EAT WHEAT

Praise For
EAT WHEAT

"John Douillard has been on the leading edge of dynamic optimal health for decades. And I have personally benefited from it. Now—he questions our obsession with gluten-free, dairy-free eating by asking the question, 'Why, after centuries of eating these foods with no problems are so many people so adversely affected by them?' His answer to that question is scientifically accurate and thought-provoking. It's because our digestion is suboptimal to begin with. And our detoxification systems are overloaded for many other reasons. Dr. Douillard has helped thousands of people cure their food intolerances by treating the cause at its root—not just the symptom. And whether or not you ever decide to consume gluten or dairy again, what you'll learn in this book is crucial to your health."

—**Christiane Northrup**, M.D., ob/gyn physician and author of
the *New York Times* bestsellers: *Goddesses Never Age: T
he Secret Prescription for Radiance, Vitality, and Wellbeing,
Women's Bodies, Women's Wisdom*, and *The Wisdom of Menopause*

"Amidst America's current gluten- and dairy-free craze, the title *Eat Wheat* may seem somewhat shocking. However, Dr. John Douillard has been a highly respected healthcare innovator for many years, and this new book may be his greatest contribution yet. His compelling evidence-based approach for safely eating wheat and dairy, will greatly ease the concerns of a rapidly growing segment of our population committed to eating healthy. For those of us who enjoy eating a well-rounded diet and believe in 'everything in moderation,' this book is a must-read."

—**Dr. Rav Ivker**, DO, ABIHM, Cofounder & Past-President, American
Board of Integrative Holistic Medicine, Past-President, American Holistic
Medical Association, and best-selling author of *Sinus Survival*

"*Eat Wheat* is clearly the most brilliant and groundbreaking dietary book in recent years that everyone should carefully read—both the lay person and the medical professional. Dr. John Douillard explodes the myths behind gluten intolerance and reveals the real culprit in our own weakened digestive systems.

He exposes similar issues behind the wholesale rejection of dairy products, which like wheat, have enormous nutritional value and usage going back thousands of years. He reveals the faulty science and commercial propaganda that have turned millions of people against some of the most valuable foods in human history.

Dr. Douillard highlights the wisdom of Ayurvedic medicine and its profound insight into the role of Agni or the digestive fire, which modern medicine has not yet properly understood. He carefully explains how, by improving our digestive fire, we can increase both our food choices and promote our own positive health and vitality."

—**Dr. David Frawley**, author *Yoga and Ayurveda*, and *Ayurvedic Healing*

"What?? Could it really be true that you can eat bread again? Dr. John Douillard—a leading expert in Ayurveda, a 5,000-year-old system of holistic medicine, and one of the most brilliant physicians I've ever met—says 'Yes!' Just like the great cholesterol myth, Dr. Douillard says gluten has been wrongly targeted as the source of your digestive problems. Instead, he contends that weak digestion is the true issue. *Eat Wheat* lays out the compelling scientific evidence that supports this seemingly radical idea and shows you how the wisdom of Ayurveda can help you to not only feel better than you ever have, but also how to strengthen your digestion so much that you'll be able to enjoy your forbidden favorite food again: a mouthwatering, fresh-out-of-the-oven, steaming hot slice of bread coated with melting butter."

—**Christine Horner, M.D.**, board-certified surgeon, natural health expert and best-selling author of *Waking the Warrior Goddess* **and** *Radiant Health, Ageless Beauty*

"Combining insights from modern scientific research and the brilliant, ancient system of Ayurvedic medicine, Dr. John Douillard takes the analysis of food sensitivities deeper to get at the root causes. Ayurveda teaches that if you can't digest a particular food—even if it's packed with nutrients, organically grown, and cooked with mother's love—it can cause symptoms, even disease. *Eat Wheat* explains not just which foods cause problems, but why, and what (beyond simply avoiding them) you can do about it."

—**Timothy McCall, M.D.**, author of *Yoga as Medicine: The Yogic Prescription for Health and Healing*, Founder/Director of Yoga As Medicine Seminars and Teacher Trainings, Co-Editor of *The Principles and Practice of Yoga in Health Care*, Medical Editor for *Yoga Journal*, and creator of DrMcCall.com

"The Sanskrit word for wheat is 'godhuma.' 'Go' means the organs of the senses and 'dhuma' means to remove the cloud of perception. Wheat actually improves sensory perception, and to remove it from our diet impairs our perceptions. When we strengthen our metabolic fire, we are able to digest gluten and dairy products."

—**Vasant Lad, B.A.M.S., M.A.Sc.**, Ayurvedic Physician, author of *Ayurveda: Science of Self-Healing*, *Textbook of Ayurveda* series and more

"How is it possible that after all these years on this planet, we humans are still debating what foods are good for us and what foods are not? In this book, Dr. Douillard makes a compelling scientific argument to show that wheat and dairy are not problematic foods if consumed properly and in moderation."

—**Joshua Rosenthal**, CEO of Institute of Integrative Nutrition

"If you are one of the millions of people that have eliminated wheat and dairy from your diet, and yet you're still suffering with digestive woes and questioning why you're not feeling your best, the answers lie within the pages of this groundbreaking book. Using traditional wisdom combined with modern science, Dr. John Douillard, gets to the root cause of the wheat and dairy controversy and teaches you how to start eating delicious foods again without compromising your life or your health."

—**Andrea Beaman**, Chef/HHC/Educator

ALSO BY JOHN DOUILLARD

Books

Body, Mind, and Sport
The Mind-Body Guide to Lifelong Health, Fitness, and Your Personal Best

Perfect Health for Kids
10 Ayurvedic Health Secrets Every Parent Must Know

The 3-Season Diet
Eat the Way Nature Intended: Lose Weight, Beat Food Cravings, Get Fit

Ayurvedic Encyclopedia of Massage

The Yoga Body Diet
Slim and Sexy in 4 Weeks Without the Stress

Colorado Cleanse
14-Day Ayurvedic Digestive Detox and
Lymph Cleanse and Seasonal Cookbook

DVDs

Ayurveda for Detox
Ayurveda for Stress Relief
Ayurveda for Weight Loss

eCourses

28-Day Ayurveda Challenge
Change Your Daily Routine, Change Your Life

John Douillard's Ayurvedic Pulse Reading Course
A Technique for Self-Discovery

Transformational Awareness Technique
6 Meditations to Emotional Freedom

For details and excerpts please visit http://store.lifespa.com.
Sign up for Dr John's **Video-Newsletter**,
and he'll let you know when each new book is published.

EAT
WHEAT

A Scientific AND *Clinically-Proven Approach* TO
Safely Bringing Wheat AND *Dairy Back* INTO *Your Diet*

DR. JOHN DOUILLARD, DC, CAP

New York

EAT WHEAT

A Scientific AND *Clinically-Proven Approach* TO *Safely Bringing Wheat* AND *Dairy Back* INTO *Your Diet*

© 2017 DR. JOHN DOUILLARD, DC, CAP.

Published in New York, New York, by Morgan James Publishing. Morgan James and The Entrepreneurial Publisher are trademarks of Morgan James, LLC.
www.MorganJamesPublishing.com

The Morgan James Speakers Group can bring authors to your live event. For more information or to book an event visit The Morgan James Speakers Group at www.TheMorganJamesSpeakersGroup.com.

Shelfie

A **free** eBook edition is available with the purchase of this print book.

CLEARLY PRINT YOUR NAME ABOVE IN UPPER CASE

Instructions to claim your free eBook edition:
1. Download the Shelfie app for Android or iOS
2. Write your name in **UPPER CASE** above
3. Use the Shelfie app to submit a photo
4. Download your eBook to any device

ISBN 978-1-68350-009-4 paperback
ISBN 978-1-68350-010-0 eBook
ISBN 978-1-68350-011-7 hardcover
Library of Congress Control Number:
2016904953

Cover Design by:
Rachel Lopez
www.r2cdesign.com

Interior Design by:
Bonnie Bushman
The Whole Caboodle Graphic Design

Edited by:
Karis Samson, Vonalda Utterback, and Jen Freed

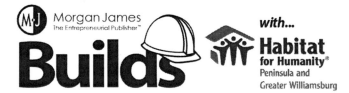

Morgan James
The Entrepreneurial Publisher™
Builds

with...
Habitat for Humanity®
Peninsula and
Greater Williamsburg

In an effort to support local communities, raise awareness and funds, Morgan James Publishing donates a percentage of all book sales for the life of each book to Habitat for Humanity Peninsula and Greater Williamsburg.

Get involved today! Visit
www.MorganJamesBuilds.com

DEDICATION

This book is dedicated to the thousands of my patients who trusted me to help them heal themselves. Their journeys made it possible to write this book.

TABLE OF CONTENTS

SUCCESS STORIES

"Dr. John Douillard helped me discover I was, in fact, never allergic to wheat. My issue was what wheat I was eating - and what it was combined with. I learned to pay attention to all the processing in the wheat products I was eating. I don't even think about wheat now, I just eat good, and real food." —**Kobe**[1]

"I have had digestion issues from birth and also lots of anxiety. This is the first time in my life that I have felt true peace in my gut, heart and head, all at the same time. Thank you, thank you, thank you!!!!!!!" —**Felicity**

"I feel like my body is digesting the food better. I have had two normal bowel movements a day, plus. I usually have one first [thing] in the morning, smaller one after breakfast, and a larger one after dinner. I use to have only one. So, my belly is flatter. I feel more sensitive to food, knowing better when to stop and desiring more vegetables and beans and rice vs meat." —**Adam**

---

1   All names of patients have been changed throughout this book to protect their privacy, and all patients have given permission to share the story of their health journey in this book. Testimonials are not claimed to represent typical results. All testimonials are real patients, and may not reflect the typical user's experience, and are not intended to represent or guarantee that anyone will achieve the same or similar results. Every person has unique experiences, exercise habits, eating habits, and applies the information in a different way. Thus, the experiences that we share from other people may not reflect the typical users' experience. However, these results are meant as a showcase of what some of Dr. John's patients have achieved. Weight Loss is not a goal of this program but on average users could expect to lose 0 to 5 pounds.

"I do feel my digestive strength has improved and I have a greater understanding [of] how the body works and the effects of emotions on the digestive system." —**Aldric**

"My husband and I went out for the "test drive" meal where we ate rich, fried, delicious foods—but this time? No problems! I was happy and, I must admit, a little bit surprised. :)" —**Judith**

"I lost 10 pounds, and 2 weeks later, I was still 7 or 8 lbs down—so it seems I have stabilized at 7 or 8 lbs lower." —**Anton**

"My digestion is so much better. Eliminating MUCH better, feeling much better overall. Morning stomach aches seemed to have dissipated for the most part." —**Lina**

"I have continued to apply what I have learned from that cleanse and still am conscious of my digestive strength. While it has taken longer than a few weeks, I am now able to digest what I was able to digest 7 years ago, or before I experienced a very stressful and emotionally abusive environment for over a year. To give you an example as to what I couldn't eat, besides the wheat and dairy, even fruit would cause me problems because of the natural sugars. Alcohol and any junk food or sweet food also obviously caused problems. I was basically living on rice and veggies. The knowledge I gained helped me understand that I could restore my digestive strength and how I could do it, and I have. While I thought when I was sick I would keep a healthy diet when I got better, I am now eating chips and chocolate, drinking any alcohol and having takeaways whenever I like with no problems. I am once again enjoying food. I guess I am making up for the years I couldn't. And just in case that sounds really bad, I am a healthy 80kgs, 6 feet tall and leading a very active lifestyle." —**Edward**

"I lost 6 lbs and the most notable result is vastly improved digestion—not a hint of heartburn, etc. I had really accepted digestion issues as a part of aging (I'm 56). Now, I really believe what Dr. John says: most of us can have the digestive strength of a teenager with a little attention." —**Katerina**

"I no longer suffer from seasonal allergies and I no longer have bloating and abdominal discomfort from eating garlic. Thank you! I am very slowly introducing gluten dairy sugar caffeine—I have been nicely attuned to seasonal eating for the last 3 years—Thank You again!" —**Elena**

"My digestive fire was definitely improved and has remained strong. I would add that my immunity was noticeably stronger after the first Colorado Cleanse I did." —**Bernard**

"I am completely off of fiber supplements. I hadn't been regular without them for more years than I care to count. Now my digestion is working perfectly, and I am thrilled."—**Anastasia**

"My digestion is the best it has been for years. Over time the changes in my health have been profound. Eventually, my craving for sugar fell away; not enjoyment of sugar, but I very seldom have any. For about a year, I stopped eating wheat and gluten to see how that felt. I didn't miss it, and then concluded I could eat it without it being poison, like when my 95-year-old mother takes me for a slice of her favorite pizza. Without sugar, the aches and pains of decades have fallen away dramatically; it is night and day! I eat yoghurt and have been known in winter to consume local grass-fed cream as a major food group. Of course I follow Doctor John in many other ways and am sincerely grateful. Meanwhile, I have become used to good, regular, often perfect digestion, so know when things go off something new is at work: a sub-clinical virus, or stress, which I then adjust to fix. Thanks to you all at Lifespa. I need to become a poet to truly express my gratitude." —**Sebastian**

"I am now able to eat Greek yogurt and a little cheese without gastric distress (lactose intolerant)." —**Iva**

"Lost 8 lbs. and feel so much cleaner, and I can trust my stomach and digestion now." —**Emily**

"My digestion was completely reset, too many small & welcome changes to mention." —**Matilda**

"We truly appreciate Dr. John for what I believe is his brilliant impartation of applying ancient Ayurveda to our food-sick culture. You have helped our whole family so much, especially with digestive issues and overcoming fatigue." —**Rachel**

"I was able to re-introduce dairy to my diet in small amounts." —**Max**

"The feeling of always carrying a cinder block in my lower abdomen has gone." —**Antonio**

"My belly is not bloated and swollen like I'm 6 months pregnant. I feel so much better!!" —**Paula**

"I dabbled in small amounts of dairy the last few weeks to see if my gut healed well enough with no gas or bloating... a taste of my husband's gelato, the home made grits at my fav restaurant... I'm digesting faster and am regular again." —**Michael**

"I am now able to digest small amounts of dairy, which I had lost the ability to do before." —**Tristan**

"It feels like my digestive system is reset, yeah!" —**Leo**

"My digestion is much better, no bloating after meals!!" —**Eva**

"I had pizza the other day and didn't get bloated or gassy!" —**Darius**

"I used to follow a vegetarian diet and then a vegan diet. After suffering lots of health issues from starches/grains I ended up going back to eating animal products and flesh which has been very difficult for me. Now I've been handling starches and grains better, still not completely without issue but much better." —**Brendan**

"I was mostly surprised that my belly-bloat (held since my last pregnancy 23 years ago) and puffiness around my eyes has really diminished." —**Dana**

"I was delighted to discover that I could finally eat beans and legumes without adverse effects (ie: terrible gas pains and bloating) and that my elimination issues (constipation or runs) are completely rectified." —**Nadia**

"I'm experiencing less acid indigestion and have not had to take any meds for it." —**Carolina**

"My digestion has improved exponentially, which I am so grateful for." —**Jeanne**

"I have maintained my healthy digestion and weight and feel great overall!" —**Cristina**

ACKNOWLEDGEMENTS

I would like to thank my editor, writing and research assistant Karis Samson who took this project on as if it were her very own. Her love, wisdom, attention and brilliance shines through on every page. I am forever grateful to Karis and it has been an honor to work with her. In the final weeks, I am deeply grateful for Vonalda Utterback whose professional editing skills have shaped *Eat Wheat* into what I believe to be a powerful message that will change the way we eat—forever.

I would like to thank my entire staff who inspire me week in and week out to bridge the gap between modern science and the ancient wisdom of Ayurveda. In particular, I would like to thank my daughter, boss and office manager, Janaki, who was the project manager for this book and carried every detail of the *Eat Wheat* ball from beginning to end. Jen Freed, whose dedication to LifeSpa is felt in every article she edits, and for her scrubbing the typos and copy-editing in *Eat Wheat* I am beyond grateful. Tauna Houghton who mocked up the initial jacket cover that convinced us all that this book would become a bestseller. Erica Illingworth for her creative genius and my sounding board for sanity, as well as Anna, Chelsea, Joe, Tony and Danielle for their everyday belief and dedication for what we do at LifeSpa. Thank you all.

I would like to thank my wife, Ginger, who spent countless hours sharing her wisdom as my research assistant, editor, troubleshooter, designer, writer and inspiration.

Finally, I would like to thank Karen Anderson at Morgan James for instantly understanding the *Eat Wheat* message and inspiring me to join the Morgan James family.

MEDICAL DISCLAIMER

Throughout this book, I will be advocating the seasonal reintroduction of hard-to-digest foods into your diet, enabled through balancing, and strengthening the digestive system. However, if you have a diagnosed condition from your primary care physician contraindicating these foods, please avoid them.

For instance, those with celiac disease should avoid gluten, and those with severe and/or life-threatening allergies to dairy should avoid dairy, etc. If you have one of these conditions, please follow the instructions of your primary care physician, as ingesting these foods can be dangerous for your health in these situations.

All material provided in this book is intended for informational and/ or educational purposes only. Speak with your medical doctor regarding the applicability of any opinions or recommendations with respect to your symptoms or medical condition. The instructions and advice presented here are in no way intended as medical advice or as a substitute for medical counseling. The information in this book should be used in conjunction with the guidance and care of your physician.

Consult with your physician before beginning this program as you would any detox, weight loss, or weight maintenance program. Your physician should be aware of all medical conditions that you may have as well as the medications and supplements you are taking.

If you are pregnant, on diuretics or diabetes medication, have liver or gallbladder concerns, a diagnosed disease, or if you are taking any medications, you should proceed only under a doctor's supervision.

You must be at least 16 years of age or older to follow the recommendations in this book. These recommendations are not intended for or applicable to those under the age of 16.

The statements made in this book have not been evaluated by the U.S. Food and Drug Administration. The contents of this book are not intended to diagnose, treat, cure or prevent any disease.

INTRODUCTION

Eating gluten- and dairy-free has taken the health food industry by storm. Food manufacturers are realizing that unless they offer a gluten-free version of their product, it is increasingly difficult to be competitive. Studies show that within a single year, as many as 100 million Americans consume gluten-free products.[1] Non-dairy foods and milk substitutes have become more common: In 2015, the U.S. dairy alternatives market was worth 2.09 billion, and growing.[2]

I invite you to join me in exploring the cause of food sensitivities and the trending gluten-free and dairy-free diets that often accompany such sensitivities. Are these types of elimination diets really necessary?

I wrote this book because, for 30 years, I have been clinically able to help my patients start eating wheat, dairy and other hard-to-digest foods again, simply by rebooting the strength of their digestive system and helping them navigate around the highly processed versions of these foods.

The "grain brain" phenomenon—namely, the notion that gluten negatively affects our brains and our health and should thus be avoided[3]—has now been challenged by a recent scientific discovery that explains the reaction many people have to wheat and dairy. Researchers have found lymphatic vessels in the brain and central nervous system (CNS) that drain directly into the body's main lymphatic system. The discovery is groundbreaking; as previously, science did not know these lymphatic vessels even existed. The science shows that numerous toxins—including beta-amyloid plaques, which are linked to Alzheimer's disease[4]—are drained from the brain through the brain's lymphatic channels while we sleep.[5]

This research is so compelling because it suggests that commonly, in the case of "grain brain"[3] and other food intolerance health issues, these brain and CNS lymphatics as well as other lymph channels may be congested, and thus cannot flow or drain toxins out of our systems properly. Let's follow this to its logical conclusion: Lymphatic congestion can lead to a heightened immune response resulting in inflammation in the body. Inflammation is directly linked to a host of digestive issues, food sensitivities and other health concerns.[5-19] Therefore, it's not the "grain," but the "drains" that may be the real culprit behind this food sensitivity epidemic.

A healthy lymphatic system starts with good upper digestion and a healthy intestinal tract. It is the primary circulatory system that processes both nutrients *and* toxins from the intestines.[16] When the ability to digest certain proteins breaks down—which is all too common today in our stressful world laden with toxins—proteins like gluten and casein from dairy, ultimately clog the lymphatic system surrounding the intestinal tract. Over time, the lymphatic system, which drains waste from every cell in the body, can become congested, leading to food intolerances that we have blamed on foods like wheat, dairy, and others.[16]

Our direct human ancestors have been eating wheat and other grains for 3.4 million years[20, 21] and early humans have been grinding wheat into flour for 30,000 years,[22] making the path to continue eating wheat in our modern times very clear: Decongest the lymphatic system, reboot digestive strength and shift our food focus away from simple sugars to good, healthy fats, along with foods in their whole, natural state.

Your digestive system is responsible for delivering nutrients as well as escorting dangerous toxins out of your body. If your digestion is weak, simply eliminating wheat or dairy from the diet is an oversimplification

of the real problem, and does not begin to address the root cause of
the issue.

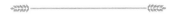

Many people spend years adjusting their diets to avoid food-related
symptoms to protect themselves from further irritation and inflammation of
the digestive tract, but this does not address the root cause. There are major
health risks involved with simply treating the symptoms of poor digestion by
removing foods from the diet. For example, if you take gluten out of the diet
when the cause of the gluten intolerance is actually weak digestion or a congested
lymphatic system then dangerous toxins can be allowed to accumulate and can
be deposited in fat cells, including the brain, for years to come.[23][27]

While you may receive symptomatic relief, simply eliminating wheat and
dairy out of your diet may give you a false sense of health and well-being. Your
inability to digest gluten or dairy—particularly if you were once able to—may
mean that you are unnecessarily being exposed to dangerous disease-producing
toxins that are not being fully digested or detoxified.

Your digestive strength is the key to a long, healthy and vital life. The choice
as to whether or not you can eat gluten or dairy should not be decided *for* you
because of weak digestion, it should be decided *by* you as a preference.

Let's stop treating symptoms, which we do oh-so-well in the West, and
finally address the urgent need to fix the root cause of our food sensitivities—the
state of our digestion.

PART I
Exploring the Cause of Wheat and Dairy Intolerance

"Start by doing what's necessary; then do what's possible; and suddenly you are doing the impossible."
—St. Francis of Assisi

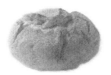

Chapter 1

FOUND GUILTY
WITHOUT A FAIR TRIAL

H as gluten been found guilty without a fair trial? It wouldn't be the first time an innocent food was given a life sentence. For example, after almost 60 years of so-called "hard science" condemning cholesterol, we now find out that the interpretation of the science was flawed and high cholesterol saturated fats, such as butter, have been officially taken off the FDA's nutrient concern list.[28]

Is it possible that we have wrongfully given gluten the boot as well, along with dairy and other commonly allergenic foods such as eggs, soy, corn, fish and nuts?

Today, there are millions of people without celiac disease or severe dairy allergies who are electing to be gluten-free and/or dairy-free, not because they are actually allergic to these foods, but because of their food sensitivities, or simply because these foods have been labeled as dietary "no-no's." It is the aim of this book to share the compelling scientific and clinical evidence that gluten—along with other specified foods, such as dairy—is often not the underlying issue in the case of digestive woes and food sensitivities.

For many, the underlying issue is actually a broken down digestive system caused by:

1. Overeating certain food groups, resulting in inflamed skin that lines the intestinal tract.
2. Making poor food choices that slowly break down digestive strength and gut health.
3. Preparing and eating certain foods at the wrong times and in the wrong ways.
4. Eating out of season.
5. Eating commercially processed bread and dairy that contains herbicides, pesticides (sometimes even genetically engineered pesticides), antibiotics, preservatives, cooked oils and growth hormones that our bodies were never designed to digest.

All of these actions compromise our digestive strength. It's no wonder so many people are no longer able to properly digest these foods!

Starting From the Top: What *Is* Gluten, Anyway?

Gluten refers to the proteins found in wheat and wheat products—including wheat berries, spelt, bulgur, durum, couscous, farina, farro, semolina, emmer, einkorn, graham, wheat bran, wheat germ, wheat starch, and KAMUT® khorasan wheat. Other common sources of gluten include triticale (a hybrid of wheat and rye), rye, barley, various forms of malt, and brewer's yeast. Oats sometimes contain gluten, but are usually gluten-free when they are specifically labeled "not contaminated by wheat." Generally speaking, gluten behaves as a glue-like element, helping foods to bind together and preserve their shape.[29-31]

A Brief History of Gluten

It's important to know that gluten is *not* the new kid on the block. There is archeological evidence of flour from wild cereal grains made in (what is now) Europe from around 30,000 years ago, during the Upper Paleolithic era.[22] And, around 10,000 years ago, with the widespread rise of farming and agriculture during the Neolithic era, bread and cereals became seasonal dietary staples.[32-34]

Contrary to what we have been led to believe, our early ancestors may have eaten much more grass, grain and wheat than previously thought, as the Ice Age forced them to venture out of the tropical rain forests into the grassland savannas, and look for new food sources.

Field studies have shown that a human can gather enough wheat berries from a field to supply enough nutrition for the entire day in just 2 hours, so why wouldn't early humans gather the easy-to-obtain grains from the grasslands as a mainstay of their diet? New findings suggest they did.[35, 36]

In the same groundbreaking report out of the University of Utah, the earliest evidence of human ancestors scavenging already-dead meat did not appear until 2.5 million years ago. Moreover, definitive evidence that humans hunted for their food does not appear until 500,000 years ago.[20, 21]

As for our direct human ancestors, this study suggests that about 3.4 million years ago, the hominin, *Australopithecus afarensis* and other human relatives ate, on average, 40 percent grasses, which included gluten-rich barley and wheat. By 1.7–2 million years ago, early humans ate 35 percent grasses and some scavenged meat from grazing animals, while another nearby hominin, *Paranthropus boisei,* was eating 75 percent grasses, including wheat.

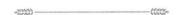

To be precise, according to the science, we should be making the case that humans have less genetic experience eating meat than we do wheat.[20, 21]

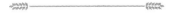

As the studies show, humans have been eating gluten for a very long time. Why is it that, suddenly, after so many thousands or millions of years of eating wheat and other glutenous grains as in-season dietary staples, eating a gluten-free diet is now one of the most prominent dietary trends?

Explaining the Gluten-Free Trend

Many people report feeling better without eating gluten. It boils down, in part, to this: If you are not able to digest gluten well, it can lead to common symptoms such as allergies, bloating, gas, belly fat, brain fog and focus issues, chronic fatigue, insomnia, autoimmune conditions, attention deficit disorder, asthma, memory loss, headaches, rashes, joint pain, digestive issues, malaise, anxiety, depression, cravings, exhaustion and, of course, weight gain.[37] No fun, right? These are all extremely valid reasons to want to avoid it.

So, you may stop eating gluten, for instance, and create a gluten-free diet based on treating the symptoms—but not the cause—of your digestive issues. This is how the rise of the popular gluten-free and other restrictive diets came to be.

I completely understand the reasoning behind why being gluten-free is such a popular choice. If you know that eating gluten doesn't make you feel good, who in their right mind would continually choose to eat it, after all? In fact, sparing your digestive tract from the ravages of undigested proteins and allergenic foods caused by weak digestion is a good strategy *in the short-term.*

I am proposing an alternative to a life sentence of restrictive diets that eliminate an entire food group. Instead, let's get to the root of the issue and heal the problem at its core and, in doing so, eliminate the symptoms caused by food intolerances. While we're at it, we will build a digestive strength that won't predispose us to susceptibility for toxin-induced chronic, degenerative diseases such as cancer and autoimmune disorders down the road.

Healing, balancing, and rebooting your digestion should allow you to once again easily digest foods like wheat and dairy. Imagine enjoying an ice cream or a delicious pastry, on occasion, without paying a painful price shortly thereafter. In this book, I will show you how to do exactly that, and explain why it is so crucially important to our health and well-being to have an optimally functioning digestive system.

As a strong digestive system is required to break down and eliminate ingested environmental chemicals and pollutants—which are, yes, even on your organic produce[38]—healing the digestive system is more important now than ever before. A new EPA analysis reports that almost 4 billion pounds of chemicals—62 million of them carcinogenic—are released into the environment each year in the U.S. alone.[39]

If you cannot tolerate wheat and dairy now, but once could, or you have found yourself slowly removing foods from your diet over the years, then this may be a sign that your ability to both digest and detoxify is compromised, which also puts you at risk for unnecessary exposure to the dangerous chemicals and toxins in our environment.

The Prevalence of Gluten Sensitivity

Estimates show that for every person with celiac disease (approximately 0.5–1 percent of the U.S. population), there are at least 6–7 people with gluten sensitivity,[40] which would put the approximate number of people with gluten sensitivities upwards of 3–7 percent of the population. With the current U.S. population in 2015 at around 322 million people and counting,[41] that would mean there are upwards of anywhere between 9.66–22.54 million people in the U.S. with gluten sensitivities. That's a lot of people who are sensitive to gluten, and these numbers do not begin to reflect those with intolerances to dairy and other hard-to-digest foods.

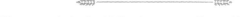

60–70 million people in the U.S. alone are affected by digestive diseases and issues.[42] These are staggering statistics and, in my opinion, this prevalence of digestive issues can be decreased dramatically through strengthening and balancing our digestive system, using time-tested strategies that have been working in traditional cultures for thousands of years.

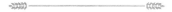

Let's heal your digestive system! To accomplish this, I will be giving you evidence-based natural healthcare strategies in combination with wisdom from India's 5,000-year-old traditional healthcare science, Ayurvedic medicine, as well as clinically proven strategies from more than 30 years in my natural medicine practice.

Some Facts, For Starters

While this subject is hotly debated, there is good science suggesting the original wild wheat, with less exposure to the environmental toxins of our modern world, may have had gluten levels that reached almost twice the amount of gluten in today's wheat![32, 43] Suggesting that, based on gluten levels alone, the original wild wheat was a much *harder* grain to digest compared to today's wheat.

When researchers compared the gliadin components of gluten from 2 ancient wheat varieties, Kamut and Graziella Ra with modern varieties, the ancient wheats had total gliadin and alpha-gliadin levels that were almost twice as high as the modern wheat varieties. Alpha-gliadin is considered the indigestible toxic form of wheat that is linked to many of the gluten sensitivity symptoms.[32, 43]

In another study, inflammation markers were measured on 22 people who ate either the ancient wheat, Kamut, or a modern wheat strain for 8 weeks. The group that ate the Kamut, where they found almost twice the amount of toxic gliadins in the previous study, saw a more than 2 times reduction in the common inflammatory markers associated with gluten sensitivity compared to the group that ate the modern wheat. How could the wheat with the highest toxic gliadin levels be almost twice as anti-inflammatory as the wheat with the least amount of gluten and gliadins?[44]

In that same study, the Kamut lowered total cholesterol, fasting blood sugar and increased magnesium and potassium levels in the blood compared to the modern wheat, suggesting that the ancient wheats are a much better choice, even though they may have more gluten and gliadins.[44] I agree.

Here is the scenario we find ourselves in: We are blaming gluten and it's gliadins as the cause of our digestive imbalances, yet ancient wheat may have had almost twice the gluten that modern wheat does,[32, 43] and people have been eating gluten for millions of years.[20, 21] How could it be that suddenly gluten has become such an issue? How could our modern gluten be solely responsible for the recent litany of health concerns and food sensitivities?

Glutenous grains are processed and prepared much differently in our modern day than they used to be. There are actually marked differences that would have made digesting ancient wheat, even with almost 2 times more gluten than modern wheat,[32, 43] easier to digest. For example, studies also show ancient wheat had more antioxidants than modern wheat, which may have offset its heightened gluten levels.[45, 46] The good news is that ancient wheats are readily available in the marketplace. I'll tell you where in Chapter 7.

In the late 19th century, technology was introduced that allowed us to process mass amounts of grains and separate the whole grain into various components. The nutrient-dense bran and germ were stripped away from the carb-rich endosperm (the part we now eat), which spikes our blood sugar without the nutrient boost.[47]

Ancient grain varieties were also traditionally prepared differently. They were often soaked, sprouted, and fermented before consumption, rendering them easier to digest and increasing their nutritional value. These practices, which are also in use today, can almost completely break down gluten, boost mineral content, increase levels of amino acids like lysine that make nutrients more easily absorbed and break down anti-nutrients like phytic acid.[47-49]

Certain studies show that although there has been an increase in celiac-based gluten intolerance in the second half of the 20th century,[32] there is no evidence that this rise is due to an increase of the gluten content in wheat. In fact, according to a 2013 study in the *Journal of Agriculture and Food Chemistry*, the gluten content in wheat during the 20th and 21st century has been relatively stable since wheat processing began in the late 19th century, and the average consumption of wheat flour in America has decreased by a whopping 86 pounds per person per year from the year 1900–2008.[32]

If the gluten content in wheat hasn't increased and the amount of wheat we are consuming has decreased, then we need to question how the recent rise in non-celiac gluten sensitivity (NCGS) cases could be caused by gluten. Most of my patients who stop eating gluten feel better only for a short time before the symptoms start to creep back, so again, how could it be just the gluten? Could we be missing something like we did with the 60-year cholesterol faux pas? The science will show that there are a handful of factors that are contributing to the current prevalence of gluten sensitivity, and if we stop to fix the cause of these problems, instead of just eliminating wheat altogether, most people will find that they can begin to enjoy eating wheat again.

Your Digestion on Gluten and Casein

Here is what we know: Both gluten and the casein in dairy require a strong and healthy digestive system to assimilate properly.

Stress, environmental toxins, processed foods, and a host of other factors have weakened our digestive strength, forcing many people to move from one restrictive diet to the next in an attempt to find the right diet for them—one where they can digest without issue. For years, patients on elimination diets find themselves complaining that there is nothing left that they can eat. I believe we can do better than that.

Many people, including holistic doctors and a growing number of medical doctors, have figured out that if they take away the "big three": Wheat, dairy, and rich, fatty or greasy foods, most everyone feels better. The thought is that if these foods can cause digestive trouble, they must be bad. However, if you could handle these foods when you were younger—not to mention the thousands of years of genetics we've inherited from our ancestors, who digested these foods just fine—*perhaps you have simply lost the ability to properly digest these foods.* The good news is that it's possible to *regain* the ability to digest hard-to-digest foods, even in their over-processed state—in small amounts.

Toxins and Sugar: Guilty as Charged

Early farmers who first domesticated wheat selected seeds that were larger and easier to remove when threshing. The larger the wheat seed, the more starch (sugar) and less protein the grain had. Since the gluten content in wheat is proportional to the protein content, ancient domesticated wheat gradually increased in sugar content while decreasing in gluten, gliadins and protein.[32]

As wheat became increasingly hybridized and processed, the glycemic index (how quickly a food breaks down and enters the bloodstream, creating a rise in blood sugar) of commercialized wheat products spiked.[50] For example, a slice of processed white bread or large dinner roll is about a 70 on the glycemic scale, while a slice of 100 percent stone-ground whole wheat or pumpernickel rates in at about 55.

The famed "wheat belly" is better termed "sugar belly" as many of the wheat sensitivities and studies linking gluten to these health concerns are more a result of excess sugar. Refined carbohydrates, such as processed white bread, quickly convert to sugar in the bloodstream.

This explosion of sugar from a high glycemic diet can cause every single symptom we have that is currently linked to gluten. In fact, much of the science supporting the grain brain theory, which links wheat to an increased risk of dementia, was based on the effect of sugar on the brain rather than the wheat itself. The theory suggested that wheat (and all grains for that matter) is the cause of high blood sugar and, thus, the smoking gun for Alzheimer's disease. This theory is challenged by a number of studies that show wheat actually *lowering* blood sugar[145-148] and *reducing* the risk of Alzheimer's.[51-56] Have we once again condemned an innocent grain, like we did with cholesterol, to the dangerous foods list, based on a flawed interpretation of the science?

I have the highest respect for Dr. Perlmutter, the author of *Grain Brain,* and his case is spot-on when we are talking about sugar and overeating highly processed, refined grains. Let me help you navigate around these issues and still enjoy your daily bread.

The hybridization of our food—as well as genetic modifications and toxins—has far-reaching implications upon our blood sugar, the digestibility of our food, and our health as a whole.

For instance, when gliadin (a protein found in wheat) is not digested completely, it may increase gut permeability, which makes the digestive system more susceptible to having trouble with hard-to-digest proteins.[57] Gliadin also affects our body's zonulin levels. Zonulin is a molecule that regulates our intercellular tight junctions, meaning that if our zonulin levels are deregulated, this can predispose us to the possibility of proteins from food passing through intestinal junctions into the blood and lymph, *where they don't belong*, predisposing us to issues like leaky gut syndrome and inflammation.[57, 58] But wait... we just read a study that high gliadin levels in wheat can actually reduce inflammation.

Even more confusing are the studies that high levels of wheat lectins called WGA (wheat germ agglutinin) found in wheat are linked to a host of health issues including inflammation, disruption of our digestive health and deregulated immune responses.[59]

Lectins are found in all grains, even non-gluten grains like rice and beans and even potatoes and tomatoes, which would condemn all these foods as some experts do. But in a 1999 study in the prestigious *British Medical Journal*, lectins are blocked by naturally-occurring sugars in the intestinal tract.

As we will see in Chapter 2 and 3, the science alone is confusing. The more we learn about how we digest wheat it seems, the less we know.

The unfortunate fact is that there are toxins in the environment, and thus in our food supply, that are extremely difficult to avoid. Studies tell us that these toxins can change the proteins in wheat[60, 61] and wreak havoc on the helpful enzymes in our bodies that break down gluten and other hard-to-digest proteins.[62]

The good news: We have the ability to detoxify the toxins in foods, but it requires a strong digestive system.[63] Remember, the very same channels that help us digest foods like wheat and dairy are used by the body to detoxify environmental toxins.

So, while you may do your best to eat healthy, non-processed foods, it is my mission to help you learn how to boost your digestive *and* detoxification potential. It is your birthright to live a long, healthy, happy life, break bread and enjoy a freshly baked slice of bread with butter.

Preservatives and Oils

Imagine not washing the grease off of your stove for the past 20 years. Most store-bought breads, unlike traditional artisan breads, are cooked with preservatives and oils that are difficult to digest and can congest the liver. This is because most oils oxidize or become damaged when heated, rendering them very difficult to digest. The result, over time, is thick or sluggish bile in the digestive process. This matters because bile regulates the hydrochloric acid (HCl) in the stomach, the digestive enzymes of the pancreas and duodenum, and the ability to process fats. To properly digest gluten, we need the coordinated effort of all these digestive processes and microbes working optimally to finish the job.

Tip: Check the labels on your bread to avoid breads with oils, or ask your local bakery for an ingredient list of their unlabeled bread.

Wheat Overload

Part of the problem is that we, as a culture, have overshot the wheat and gluten runway. The typical American diet has included eating wheat with every meal for the past 40–50 years. We have overeaten wheat in a *major* way.

Wheat is a cool climate grain that used to be harvested only once a year—in the fall, to be eaten in the winter. Wheat is not a crop that is naturally available year-round. And yet, we've been eating it for every meal, year-round, for decades!

For example, the original einkorn wheat became fully ripe in October, right before the winter rains. The ripe grain would fall to the ground and lie dormant all winter until spring, when the warmer temperatures and rain would help germinate and sprout the grain. Because of the ability for wheat to store well, it's a grain that can be gathered in the fall and last through the winter as a sustainable food. Nature always seems to deliver the foods we need most, at the right time of year.[64]

Eating wheat, a grain designed by nature to be eaten in the fall to help prepare for winter, was simply never meant to be eaten 3 times a day for 12 months of the year, every year, for a lifetime.

To make matters worse, in 1980, the Reagan administration subsidized the growth of wheat and corn (another hard-to-digest food) for pennies on the dollar, to keep prices down.[65] With such artificially low prices, the result was a dangerous shift in the American diet towards eating our "daily bread," 3–4 times a day, something very new for humans. To keep up with the demand, bread was processed and preserved in such a way that rendered it virtually indigestible. Today, instead of bread going bad in a few days, it can sit on a shelf for weeks without spoiling.

We know that microbes are what cause food to spoil, and that traditional artisan breads had a very short shelf life. When preservative-laden store-bought bread lasts weeks before spoiling, that means the microbes aren't eating it. 90 percent of the cells in the human body are microbial cells and these microbes do the heavy lifting for all our digestive processes including breaking down gluten.[66] If the microbes won't eat the bread that's been in your cupboard for weeks, we can't expect the same microbes to digest that bread inside your belly.

On top of that, with the subsidization of corn, high-fructose corn syrup was then incorporated into popular bread company's recipes, either replacing or in addition to sugar, making bread sweeter, but more toxic, addictive and even harder to digest.

Solution: Wheat in Season

According to our circadian rhythms—and thousands of years of ancient wisdom—eating and living in sync with the changing seasons is of utmost importance for supporting optimal health and well-being. After all, we humans are part of nature and are not exempt from its cycles.

For instance, in nature, diet changes dramatically from season to season and, like an artist's palette, the microbes needed to digest each season's harvest thrive with each seasonal cue; the woody brown branches and barks of winter are a prelude to the bright greens of spring and the golden acorns of fall.

Microbes suited to digest the soft leaves and bitter roots abounding in springtime vanish by summer, while a new population of microbes that digest the tough wood fibers and heavier foods of winter replaces microbes that feed on the juicy fruits and flavorful greens of summer.

Certain digestive enzymes like amylase increase during the winter months in humans, making the fall-harvested wheat much easier to digest in the winter months.[85] A lack of amylase (which is required to digest wheat) is linked to wheat allergies and baker's asthma.[67] This happens when we eat wheat out of season, say in the spring or summer.

As we will see, nature harvests heavier, denser and harder-to-digest foods like wheat, dairy, roots, nuts and seeds in the winter, which require more digestive strength than the light, leafy greens of the summer do.

Solution: Fermentation

Speaking of living in harmony with the cycles of nature, it is common knowledge that our ancestors figured out how to ferment their vegetables to help preserve them through the winter. Not only does fermenting preserve the food, it creates digestive-boosting microbes needed to digest the heavy and dense foods of the fall—the benefits of the winter harvest!

Fermented vegetables are very acidic and thus heat the body, which helped our relatives endure many long, cold winters.

In addition, the process for fermenting veggies is called *lactic acid fermentation*, which releases a host of *Lactobacillus bacteria* that have been shown to break down the hard-to-digest gliadin portions of the gluten protein molecule—the proline-rich epitopes that I mentioned earlier.[68, 69]

It's interesting how nature gave us gluten in the winter, and to make sure we digested it well, fermentation gave our digestive systems a naturally-occurring boost in wheat-digesting enzymes.[70]

Solution: A Boost from Probiotics

Today, many people are convinced that probiotics are the answer to all kinds of health woes. When I first went into practice in 1984, I used probiotics regularly with my patients. It didn't take long before I realized that I was only offering symptomatic relief. People felt better while on them and then quickly became dependent. As soon as they stopped taking them, the symptoms returned. The vast majority of the probiotics on the market today are made with fragile, lactic-based organisms, making them transient in nature. According to current knowledge, we will need to take a probiotic every day for the rest of our lives. This kind of dependency on a pill never sat well with me, and I hope makes no sense to you either.

The reality is that your ability to digest wheat properly is totally dependent upon the efficiency of your digestion, a healthy intestinal tract, and the right gluten-digesting microbes. Once these three problems are solved, the right kind of probiotic, taken short-term, can help you digest wheat and dairy once again. The key to probiotics, or any supplement for that matter, is self-sufficiency: You get on them, get better, and then get off them. For years I have sought to bring the digestive system back into balance rather than just give symptomatic relief, and to that end, I have been in search of strains of probiotics that were *colonizing* rather than *transient* in nature. I'm happy to report that researchers have recently discovered strains of colonizing probiotics that actually adhere to the gut wall and become permanent residents, setting the stage to rebuild a microbiome that has adapted over millions of years to digest wheat.

New studies show that there are beneficial bacteria in the gut that help us digest gluten. There are also certain probiotic supplements (such as *Lactobacillus plantarum* and *Bifidobacterium lactis*) that help break down and digest the gliadin proline-rich epitopes, which are the hard-to-digest part of the gluten protein molecule.[68, 69, 71] Probiotics have also been shown to protect the intestinal wall by disallowing the undigested gluten molecule to penetrate the gut wall, thus protecting against leaky gut syndrome.[72]

Note: See Chapter 8 for the best colonizing strains of gluten-digesting probiotics for optimal gut health.

Help Me Boost My Digestion!

Let's recap with 6 quick tips to get you started on your path to good digestion.

- **Tip 1:** Begin by taking a cue from our ancestors and adding a quality probiotic with the strains mentioned above to your diet, which you can get through fermented foods, or in capsulated probiotic form.
- **Tip 2:** Eat gluten and dairy seasonally. Consider reducing or avoiding these foods in the spring, have a small amount of them in the summer, and enjoy them a bit more in the fall and winter. The cold months are when these foods become naturally available with the season's harvest, just as nature intended.

- **Tip 3:** Eat your largest meal at mid-day with heavy foods like wheat and dairy when the digestive fire is stronger. It is best to avoid heavy meals, wheat, dairy and starchy carbs at night, as the digestive fire is less strong in the evening.

- **Tip 4:** Grow your own food if you are able. If not, buy from local farmer's markets or join a Community Supported Farm (CSA). Many small companies are popping up, such as Door to Door Organics, who deliver fresh organic veggies to your door. Eat as much organic and non-processed foods as you can. Conventional foods that have been sprayed with pesticides and herbicides not only contain toxins, but also lack the beneficial microbes required to digest wheat and dairy. This could be the reason the Western microbiome is so lacking in microbial diversity compared to the rest of the world,[73-75] and reason enough why many are experiencing gluten sensitivity. Think of seasonal organic foods as your connection to the seasonal changes of the digestive microbes that make up 90 percent of the cells in the human body and do the heavy lifting for just about every function in the human body.[66]

 Tip: To learn more about CSAs and to locate one near you, go to http://www.localharvest.org/csa/

- **Tip 5:** Eating organic, slow fermented sourdough bread with no preservatives or oils is a great option over other breads. The fermented culture of lactic acid and probiotic strains used to make sourdough actually help to break down gluten and, according to some studies, even render the bread gluten-free.[49, 68, 76, 77] (More in Chapter 7.)

- **Tip 6:** Even better, try your hand at baking your own bread. Use fermented wheat and bake it by hand or use a bread maker. It's fun, satisfying, and easy! (Learn how to make your own healthy, homemade sourdough bread with 2 traditional recipes found in Appendix B.) Kids love the alchemy of baking, so make it a family affair!

Note: *If you are gluten and diary intolerant then avoid these foods until we reboot your digestive strength in Part II.*

Memories of Hot, Fresh Bread

When I was a child, my dad used to take me to a local bakery. Before even making it inside, the irresistible scent of freshly baked bread would hit our noses. He'd grab a fresh baguette and rip it in half to split it with me as we drove away. Still warm from the oven, I remember holding it to my cheeks between bites. This was a special time for us, and a memory I'll never forget. I'm sure many of you have memories of delicious bakery items or pastas that have stuck with you because it was a precious shared life experience.

Looking Ahead

Breaking bread with someone is fundamental human experience of trust, sharing and love. This is something I feel strongly that we shouldn't give up on without a fight. And for those of you who have gone gluten-free, I'm not trying to marginalize the effort it takes to make that transition—I know it's difficult. Rather, what I'm trying to say is, let's not be satisfied with the Band-Aid diagnosis of a food elimination diet when you may truly be able to have your bread and eat it too!

In Chapter 2, I will explore the science on both sides of the gluten aisle. You will be surprised to see how much unsung science there is touting the health benefits of wheat.

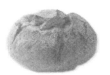

WHEAT: THE SCIENCE
TOUTING ITS BENEFITS

A s I discussed in the previous chapter, there is actually a lot of science—albeit less publicized but equally valid—showing how wheat is and has been a health-promoting staple of human's winter diet for thousands of years.

I want to be clear that I am *not* advocating eating bucketloads of wheat all of the time. Many people do feel better without it, and it is completely valid to choose to avoid gluten. What I *am* saying is that with the right kind, in the right amount, at the right time, and with strong digestion, wheat, like all foods, has a purpose with clear health benefits. Let's just make sure, before you eliminate gluten from your diet forever, that you're not putting yourself at risk for future health concerns by eliminating what causes your symptoms rather than targeting the core of the issue—weak digestion.

Remember, foods containing gluten are not an accident of nature, and humans have been eating wheat for millions of years[20, 21] for good reason. Let's explore the compelling modern science supporting its many unsung health benefits.

- **Gluten-free Science:** Ancient humans rarely or ever ate wheat or grain as part of their diet.[3]
- ***Eat Wheat!* Science:** Our ancestors hunted, but they also gathered.[78-80] They didn't have refrigerators or fancy foods imported from across the world. They ate what was available to them from nature, season to season.[81, 82] Depending on the season, the bounty our ancestors gathered from nature included grains, roots, fruits, vegetables, and other starches as staples of their diet. Early hominins ate glutenous grasses like wheat for millions of years[3,4] and, as I mentioned earlier, there is evidence of grain-based flour being made 30,000 years ago,[22] as well as a prevalence of breads and cereals as dietary staples with the rise of the agricultural Neolithic age 10,000 years ago.[32-34] Not only does gluten have an extensive track record through the ages as a dietary staple, but most research suggests that a plant-based diet rich in vegetables, fruits, and grains—not exclusive of gluten—can decrease the risk of chronic disease.[78, 82-84]
- **Gluten-free Science:** A gluten-free diet boosts immunity and gut health.
- ***Eat Wheat!* Science:** A recent study with 10 healthy adults on a gluten-free diet for 1 month showed a *decrease* in beneficial gut bacteria and an *increase* of unhealthy gut bacteria in study participants. They also saw a significant *decrease* in functioning of the immune system.

    It turns out that the fiber and carbohydrates in grains, like wheat, feed healthy "immunity-boosting" microbes in the gut. Taking gluten out of the diet actually disturbed the delicate microbial environment of the gut, which likely developed over millions of years of eating wheat.[85]

- **Gluten-free Science:** Eating gluten results in weight gain and obesity.[3]
- ***Eat Wheat!* Science:** According to Mayo Clinic's gluten expert, Joseph Murray, MD, there is no evidence that a gluten-free diet affects weight loss. Murray explains that most people on a gluten-free diet simply tend not to eat as much food in general, and thus lose weight.[86]

    Another study, performed by the Harvard Medical School and Brigham and Women's Hospital, published in the *American Journal of Clinical Nutrition,* found that women who ate more whole grains weighed less than those who ate less whole grains, while those eating more fiber from whole grains were 49 percent less likely to gain weight than those who ate more refined grain products.[87, 88]

In addition, many of the healthiest cultures from around the world eat carbohydrate-based diets, including the hunter-gatherer Hadza of north-central Tanzania, the Kuna of Panama, the Kitava in the Pacific Islands, the Tukisenta in Papua New Guinea, the Okinawans, and the Greeks. Some of these cultures have diets upwards of 69 percent and even 90 percent carbohydrates, yet they are fit and lean with practically non-existent rates of neurological disorders and other modern chronic disease.[52]

Many other studies have found that a higher consumption of whole grains (including grains with gluten) is associated with a lower body mass index.[89-92]

- **Gluten-free Science:** Eating a low or no-grain diet increases longevity.[3]
- ***Eat Wheat!* Science:** Actually, eating a diet rich in whole grains, including glutenous whole grains, has been found to support both total longevity and cardiovascular longevity by keeping us healthy.[53, 93, 94] Not only that, but in many studies, a low-carb diet has been found to *decrease* longevity and *increase* our risk of imbalances such as cardiovascular disease and cancer.[95-100]
- **Gluten-free Science:** Gluten and carbs are linked to Alzheimer's disease and dementia, and it's healthier to instead focus on a diet that is high in fat, protein and low in carbs.[3]
- ***Eat Wheat!* Science:** The research at the cornerstone of this argument,[51] suggests that high glucose levels (not wheat) is a risk factor for dementia, even among individuals without diabetes.[52, 101] This research also reports that sugar, not wheat or grains, as many gluten-free experts proclaim, is associated with Alzheimer's disease and dementia.

Processed wheat has its issues, undoubtedly, but wheat should not be implicated in connection with Alzheimer's and dementia, when the science behind this argument shows that sugar is the risk factor.

- Furthermore, the Mediterranean and DASH (Dietary Approaches to Stop Hypertension) diets include substantial amounts of whole grains—including gluten, carbohydrates, dairy, and fruit, and have been scientifically shown to reduce the risk of Alzheimer's and dementia.[53-56]

- **Gluten-free Science:** Eating gluten disrupts bowel regularity and digestive health.[3]

- *Eat Wheat!* **Science:** Whole grains are rich in fiber, and fiber helps as a bulking agent in escorting your waste to the toilet, which speeds the transit time through the intestines and helps you avoid uncomfortable and unhealthful situations like constipation.[102] In one study, high-fiber wheat foods were found to increase fecal output by 33-36 percent.[103] It is common knowledge that fiber supports healthy and more regular bowel movements, and wheat, in its unrefined form, is a good source of fiber.

- **Gluten-free Science:** The phytic acid found in grains can bind with minerals and inhibit mineral absorption, which can leave us mineral deficient. The phytic acid in grains can also diminish our digestive enzymes and thus our power to digest well, and is considered an anti-nutrient.[104]

- *Eat Wheat!* **Science:** Phytic acid is non-toxic and actually holds health benefits. It contains potent antioxidants, and has been shown to reduce levels of blood sugar, cholesterol, insulin, triglycerides, and inflammation in the body.[82, 88, 105-108]

  Studies also suggest that phytic acid can help decrease rates of cancer, heart disease, obesity, Parkinson's disease, diabetes, kidney stone formation, and other chronic diseases, and has been found to support the immune system. According to medical professionals, bacteria in the digestive tract safely metabolize excess dietary phytic acid.[82, 88, 105-108] Interestingly, the probability of children being asthmatic dropped 54 percent with a high intake of whole grains and its associated phytic acid.[109]

As we will see in Chapter 7, sourdough breads and other traditional techniques like soaking, sprouting and fermenting the grains increase phytase activity which breaks down the phytic acids for those with sensitive digestive systems.

- **Gluten-free Science:** A low-carb diet can be supportive of your cardiovascular health.[110]
- *Eat Wheat!* **Science:** Perhaps, for the short term, you can live without ample amounts of carbs and avoid deleterious effects on your cardiovascular health, but many studies show that whole grains (thus a diet containing ample complex carbohydrates) have profound supportive effects on our cardiovascular health.[111, 112]

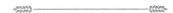

In one study published in the *American Heart Journal*, postmenopausal women who ate at least 6 servings of whole grains per week were shown to have slowed progressions of atherosclerosis and stenosis, both conditions that negatively affect circulatory pathways.[113]

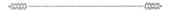

Lignan, a phytonutrient found abundantly in whole grains, is also protective against heart disease.[114] In yet another study, participants who ate a daily bowl of whole grain cereal for breakfast lowered their risk of heart failure by 29 percent.[115] High fiber through whole grains equals a healthy heart and circulatory system.

- **Gluten-free Science:** Gluten and carbohydrates contribute to the risk of breast cancer.[116]
- *Eat Wheat!* **Science:** In one study published in the *International Journal of Epidemiology,* pre-menopausal women who consumed the most fiber from whole grains reduced their risk of breast cancer by a whopping 41 percent.[88, 117]

In another study with postmenopausal women, those who ate the most fiber through cereal grains had a 50 percent reduced risk of breast cancer compared to those who ate the least amount of fiber. [88, 118] Also, whole grains were found to have high amounts of phenols and lignans, which protect against cancers such as colon and breast cancer, respectively. [114, 119]

- **Gluten-Free Science:** Eating gluten is linked with diabetes. [3]
- ***Eat Wheat!* Science:** In one recent study, metabolic syndrome—related to diabetes—was found to be 38 percent lower in those who were consuming the most cereal fiber from grains as opposed to the group eating the least amount of cereal fiber from grains. [88, 120] Diets rich in whole grains have also been scientifically associated with a 31 percent lower risk of type 2 diabetes. [121]

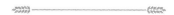

If it is not the wheat or the gluten that has been linked to blood sugar issues, it must be the refined wheat flour and processed and contaminated nature of most of the wheat we consume. Studies show repeatedly that unrefined whole wheat benefits blood sugar. [88, 120-123]

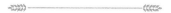

- **Gluten-free Science:** Consuming gluten is associated with depression. [3]
- ***Eat Wheat!* Science:** Diets such as the Mediterranean diet—rich in plant-based foods, including whole grains, as well as consumption of whole grain cereals, are considered the ideal diet to prevent depression. [53, 124-127] The real culprit of what has come to be known as "gluten-related depression" is likely due to over-consumption of highly processed refined white flour products and congested lymph channels that drain the brain. Poorly digested gluten can enter the lymph through the intestines and cause lymph congestion.

A recent discovery found lymphatic channels located in the brain5 that, when congested, can cause depression. Until very recently, researchers thought the brain to be devoid of lymph. Now, congested brain lymph is linked to a host of psychological concerns and inflammation.5 As we will see in Chapters 4 and 9, undigested gluten can leak through the gut and cause most gluten-related symptoms.

- **Gluten-free Science:** Gluten is linked with exacerbating the symptoms of autism.[3]
- ***Eat Wheat!* Science:** In some studies, gluten has actually been found to have no effect on those with autism, and did not exacerbate any of their symptoms.[128] In other studies, gluten has been found to affect some, but not all, subjects with autism, suggesting there are differing subgroups in the autism spectrum that respond in unique ways to gluten.[129, 130]
- **Gluten-free Science:** Gluten is linked with schizophrenia.[3]
- ***Eat Wheat!* Science:** Actually, research has shown evidence that gluten does not have a statistically significant effect upon people with schizophrenia. In one study, for example, there was no decline in clinical status or measurable inflammatory response compared to placebo when subjects with schizophrenia ate gluten.[131-133]
- **Gluten-free Science:** Gluten is associated with increased anxiety.[3]
- ***Eat Wheat!* Science:** Consumption of whole grains, including those with gluten, has been found to actually support prevention of anxiety. In fact, switching to the Mediterranean diet, with ample whole grains, has been found to have a positive effect on overall mood.[53, 127, 134-136]
- **Gluten-free Science:** Eating gluten is linked to arthritis.[3]
- ***Eat Wheat!* Science:** Whole grains have been indicated in a healthy diet for prevention of gout, associated with arthritis. For instance, multiple studies show that the grain-rich Mediterranean diet has an anti-inflammatory response on arthritic inflammation.[53, 137, 138] Furthermore, whole wheat products are a great source of betaine, a chemical compound that has been linked to decreasing inflammation in the body.[139-141]
- **Gluten-free Science:** Gluten can cause infertility.[3]
- ***Eat Wheat!* Science:** In one study, following the grain-rich Mediterranean diet helped couples conceive through in-vitro fertilization/ intracytoplasmic sperm injection therapy. Other research has shown that

women with celiac disease, an extreme form of sensitivity to gluten, have no more problems with fertility than the rest of the population.[53, 142, 143]

New research has found that there are lymphatics that drain into the reproductive system.[10] While I have not yet seen the science that links lymph congestion to infertility, it would make sense that if congested lymph channels are not draining the reproductive system properly, this could complicate matters when couples try to conceive. These lymphatic structures are newly discovered and it will take time to fully understand the role of the lymph and its relationship to infertility as well as to the disease process.

Still Confused About Gluten?

I fully acknowledge how frustrating it can be to read some of these studies about the pros of gluten if you are experiencing troublesome symptoms of gluten sensitivity. Perhaps you are still convinced that gluten is an unhealthy food. I have no doubt that, indeed, you *do* feel better in general and can even lose unwanted pounds when you stop eating gluten, dairy, and other hard-to-digest foods.

Clearly, there is science on both sides of this debate and, to reiterate, my goal is not to force wheat and dairy back into your diet. However, if weak digestion is the cause of your wheat and dairy sensitivities, for the sake of your long-term health, this weakness should be addressed. Eliminating these foods from your diet, without fixing the digestive weakness, can cause a host of health issues for years to come.

Widespread Misdiagnosis of Gluten and Dairy Intolerance

One major issue with food sensitivities is that people are being misdiagnosed en masse as having allergies to gluten, dairy and other foods, and are unnecessarily being put on lifelong restrictive diets.

For years, I have been very suspicious of allergy testing methods, because I often see patients come in with a laundry list of foods they were told to avoid for the rest of their lives. Then, 6 months later, the same allergy test would reveal a *new* list of reactive foods to avoid. Patients would come to me to help them not be so reactive to the so-called 'allergenic' foods, in part because they were running out of foods to eat based on the allergy tests.

In a study published in the *Journal of Pediatrics*, allergy skin-prick tests were found to be grossly inaccurate.[144-146] The study looked at 125 children from ages 1–9 who were diagnosed with a food allergy from a skin-prick IgE (*immunoglobulin E*) test in which a person is scratched by a needle with a protein from the suspected allergenic food. (The test is positive if the skin becomes swollen or irritated.) The researchers followed up and gave these children food challenge tests, where a reaction to a certain food was tested rather than a skin-prick allergy test, and the results were shocking. When ingesting the actual food, 93 percent of these children had no reactivity to the foods they were told to avoid for the rest of their lives.[144-146]

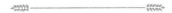

The skin test often used to diagnose gluten intolerance, has been shown by a scientific study to be *over 65 percent inaccurate*![147] Other research indicates that about 50–60 percent of the time, skin prick tests yield positive results even if you are not actually allergic to the food you're testing for tolerance to.[148] On top of that, many people are diagnosed with the celiac gene that hasn't yet been expressed, and thus people are being told, in droves, to avoid wheat.[147, 148] Studies like these illustrate the magnitude of how many people have been diagnosed with gluten intolerance that don't actually have it.

Similarly, there are widespread difficulties in diagnosing intolerance to dairy and lactose. While sugar lactose malabsorption can be measured by a lactose tolerance blood test, jejunal biopsy, or breath hydrogen test, a true intolerance can only be determined by reaction to food containing lactose, which, to complicate matters further, is often not an immediate response. This can result in a misdiagnosis of lactose intolerance.[149]

Looking Ahead

Many doctors have gotten into the habit of simply telling their patients to avoid wheat and dairy to give them symptomatic relief, without digging into the cause of their gluten or dairy intolerance. In Part II of this book, we will go straight to the root of the issue, giving you tools to heal overly sensitive and imbalanced intestinal skin and reset your digestive strength. In Chapter 3, I will discuss the science on both sides of the dairy aisle.

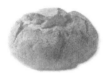

Chapter 3

DAIRY: A FOOD
AND A MEDICINE

D airy, much like gluten, has been demonized as a "taboo" or "bad" food. Similar to gluten, many folks complain that dairy causes issues such as gas, bloating, congestion, weight gain, joint pain, brain fog, and fatigue.

Some studies have linked dairy products to causing and/or exacerbating all of these complaints and more. Other studies, in contrast, have put forth compelling research linking dairy to numerous health benefits and tout it as an essential food for optimal health. With both camps citing conflicting studies, the controversy surrounding dairy can be extremely confusing, to say the least.

Many people do feel better when they eliminate dairy from their diet, and this is a completely valid reason to avoid it. However, please keep in mind that, as we previously discussed with gluten, avoiding dairy for symptomatic relief of digestive issues often masks deeper digestive issues that can cause health concerns later on.

So first, let's explore the multifarious world of dairy, shedding light on some perplexing issues and revealing an amazingly simple solution to the problems

29

associated with digesting it. Like we saw with the research on gluten, there are always two sides to every coin. So before we condemn dairy as a bad food or toxin, let's look at all sides of the research. Education is the key to making the wisest, most healthful choice.

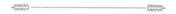

Due to lack of refrigeration and limited preservation techniques, our ancestors consumed dairy products, just like all foods, seasonally. Cows give birth in the spring when the milk is exclusively for the calf. By fall, the calf has grown big and fat enough to endure a winter, meaning there is excess dairy available for human consumption. Cold northern European winters were habitable in large part because of cows, goats and sheep. Their milk was traditionally—and still is—preserved as cheese and butter, which allowed early humans to survive harsh winters. Even today, much of Europe depends on dairy products for their nutritional needs.

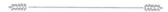

- **Dairy-free Science** Many health experts report that it is healthier to avoid dairy than to consume dairy.[150]
- *Eat Wheat!* **Science:** It might surprise you to know that studies have shown that consuming dairy has a protective effect against conditions such as stroke, diabetes, dementia, certain cancers, coronary heart disease, osteoporosis, high blood pressure, hypertension, and excessive body weight, with an overall health advantage over populations that do not consume dairy. Dairy is also an important food-based source of calcium, which is vital for our health, in adequate doses.[151-153]
- **Dairy-free Science:** Studies suggest dairy causes weight gain.[154, 155]
- *Eat Wheat!* **Science:** Actually, many studies show that dairy supports healthful weight loss and reduced body mass index.[152, 156-159] For instance, in one study, increased dairy consumption was found to be the main factor associated with weight loss in overweight adults after being involved in a lifestyle change program for 20 weeks.[156]

- **Dairy-free Science:** Studies conclude dairy is inflammatory and aggravates joint pain.[160, 161]
- *Eat Wheat!* **Science:** According to the science, dairy is linked with decreasing risk of gout, which is associated with arthritis.[162-164]
- **Dairy-free Science:** Certain sources suggest that dairy causes brain fog.[165]
- *Eat Wheat!* **Science:** There are a handful of studies showing that increased milk and dairy intake—specifically low-fat milk and dairy products—has been found to reduce risks of Alzheimer's disease, dementia, and cognitive decline.[54, 166, 167]
- **Dairy-free Science:** Dairy causes mucus and congestion.[168]
- *Eat Wheat!* **Science:** Research has shown that, in fact, consuming milk products does *not* increase the production of mucus.[169] In one study of subjects that consumed milk, people who believed that milk causes mucus actually reported more symptoms of congestion than those that didn't believe this theory, nodding to the strong power of placebo and mind over matter.[170] In another study, the placebo group who drank fake milk reported as many congestive symptoms as those who drank real milk.[171]

That said, since congestion is the most common symptom I see in my practice that appears related to dairy, let's dig in a little. According to Ayurveda, having a slightly congestive quality is actually dairy's job. Dairy is considered a heavy food, meaning it has moist, congestive qualities. It is helpful for keeping the body lubricated and insulated during cold, dry months such as fall and winter.

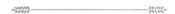

If you are experiencing over-congestive issues with dairy, there is a good chance you are either overeating it, eating a super-processed version of it (such as ultra-pasteurized), eating it out of season, or the intestinal tract is already irritated and producing excess mucus and congestion on its own.

In this case, we must reboot your digestive and intestinal health as I outline in Part II. With an optimally functioning digestive system, dairy can help to keep us in balance by providing us with a perfect balance of mucus production in our bodies when it's cold and dry outside.

- **Dairy-free Science:** The anti-dairy movement says our ancestors didn't eat dairy.[172]

- *Eat Wheat!* **Science:** Scientists have uncovered shards of pottery containing organic residues of milk from circa 7000 BC in the Near East and southeastern Europe, the earliest direct evidence of milk use to date.[173-175] In another study, researchers found DNA evidence extracted from Neolithic skeletons indicating that in 5500 BC, people in northern Europe drank milk, so it seems our ancestors *did*, in fact, eat dairy.[176] Not only that, but earthenware vessels found in England dating to 4500 BC contained milk by-products, indicating that while it's possible it was not consumed directly, milk was used in some form.[175] These studies show that humans have used dairy for a long time; it is not a new food group for us.

- Today, nearly 95 percent of the Northern European population has the gene that produces lactase, an enzyme that helps digest the lactose in dairy products.[177] According to experts, the evolution of this gene is called "lactase persistence," and it provided early Northern Europeans with a huge survival advantage.[178] Lactase persistence was so genetically advantageous that it spread and evolved quickly.[176]

- However, if your ancestors didn't live in northern Europe some 7,500 years ago, and instead, lived in eastern or southeastern Asia, where it is likely that dairy was not commonly eaten,[178] today you might be considered lactose intolerant. Not to worry, we have a fix for that! It has been used for thousands of years—it's called cheese. See the logic below.

- **Dairy-free Science:** Those with diagnosed lactose intolerance must strictly avoid all dairy.

- *Eat Wheat!* **Science:** First, let's talk about lactose intolerance. The signs and symptoms of lactose intolerance usually begin 30 minutes after eating or drinking foods that contain lactose. Common signs and symptoms include nausea, sinus congestion, abdominal cramps, bloating, gas, and loose bowels.

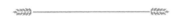

Here's the good news: Folks who are lactose intolerant can still enjoy some naturally lactose-free dairy, according to many experts. In the process of making cheese, and particularly cottage cheese, the lactose is converted to lactic acid, which is easier to digest. Even if you have determined that you have lactose intolerance, you should still be able to eat cheese.

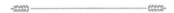

- Raw cheese is now legal in the U.S. if it ages for at least 3 months before selling it. During those 3 months, the non-pasteurized raw cheese microbes will gobble up the milk sugar as their main source of fuel, rendering the raw, aged cheese mostly devoid of any lactose. This process also predigests the casein found in dairy that is considered difficult to digest.[179] Cream and butter have zero lactose. Bring on the butter! The lactose in yogurt is mostly converted to lactic acid as well, making it tolerable for most. Skim milk still has lactose, however, so it is not a good choice for lactose intolerant individuals.
- **Dairy Science:** Dairy is a good source of calcium. Calcium is needed for strong bones.
- *Eat Wheat!* **Science:** Calcium is important for strong bones, but the biggest factor regarding calcium absorption is actually getting adequate amounts of vitamin D3. Vitamin D3 is required to carry the dietary calcium out of the gut and into the bloodstream. We primarily absorb our vitamin D3 from the sun or with supplementation. The cream portion of milk is a good supply of vitamin D3, along with the other essential fat-soluble vitamins A, E and K. Unfortunately, these vitamins are broken down in the pasteurization and homogenization process. As a result, milk is fortified with synthetic vitamins A, D2 (not D3) and calcium.

Up to 78 percent of Americans are vitamin D3-deficient.[180] It is the chronic deficiency of vitamin D3 that causes calcium deficiencies, which in turn may be linked to bone density issues. In general, milk alone does not deliver enough vitamin D3 to reach the benefits that vitamin D3 optimization provides. Vitamin D3 supplementation in the winter and regular midday sun exposure in the summer—within sensible, healthy limits to avoid sunburn—is strongly recommended for optimal health and strong bones.

- **Dairy Science:** Pasteurization and ultra-pasteurization are the gold standard for milk processing.
- *Eat Wheat!* **Science:** Pasteurization is a hotly debated topic and may be the most confusing. Pasteurization is a process that heats milk in order to kill foodborne bacteria, microbes and pathogens. While pasteurization has saved lives when dairy farms were less than sanitary, today many take issue with this process. The ultra-pasteurization of milk, in particular, is used to extend shelf life and increase profits margins. It does not make milk safer or healthier.
- By killing the bad bugs, the good bugs are also killed, along with the enzymes so desperately needed to break down the hard-to-digest proteins and fats and deliver the vitamins and minerals. Raw milk advocates, such as the Weston Price Foundation, link the pasteurization process itself to sinus congestion, heart health concerns, circulation, cholesterol issues and more.[181]

There are 3 kinds of pasteurization that you might see written on a label:

Ultra-Pasteurized
- Heats milk to 275°F for a couple of seconds
- Shelf life of 1–2 months

- Kills everything
- Avoid

Pasteurized
- Traditional process: Heats milk to 160°F for 15–20 seconds
- Shelf life of 2–3 weeks
- Preserves some good bacteria
- Try to avoid

Vat-Pasteurized
- Heats milk to 135°F for 20 minutes
- Shelf life of 7–10 days. It's still alive!
- Preserves good bacteria and many enzymes
- Best commercial choice and my recommendation

Vat-pasteurization is becoming a more popular option. It provides a guaranteed product, free of bad bacteria while preserving many of the enzymes and good bacteria because the heat is relatively low.

While many of Organic Valley's milk products are ultra-pasteurized and should be avoided, they do offer one product called "Grassmilk" which is a grass-fed, cream-on-top, non-homogenized, pasteurized, whole milk product. Kalona Supernatural brand, which also distributes nationally, offers a variety of vat-pasteurized, non-homogenized products found at natural foods markets. Many more products like this are coming, and can be found at your local health food market.

Dairy Intolerant? Try it Vat-Pasteurized
Heating milk too fast at high temperatures during conventional "flash" pasteurization will of course kill the bacteria, but also damages the casein rendering it very difficult to digest.[182, 183] However, according to Ayurveda, heating pasteurized milk slowly to just when it starts to boil will kill the bacteria and pathogens, but leave the good bacteria and the enzymes. This process is an ancient form of vat-pasteurization and will

help break down the damaged casein in pasteurized commercial milk. If you buy pasteurized milk and typically have trouble digesting it, bring it slowly to a boil, let it cool, and then drink it, and see if you digest it better.

I have numerous patients who say they have been dairy-intolerant for years who, once they try a vat-pasteurized milk, can tolerate it without a problem. Like wheat, it is often not the milk itself that is the issue; the problem is in the processing.

 Tip: Avoid ultra-pasteurized milk. If you buy pasteurized milk, heat it the Ayurvedic way. Look for vat-pasteurized milk, or better yet, choose legal, raw dairy products. For best digestibility, bring raw products to a slow boil as well.

- **Dairy Science:** Skim milk has less calories, so it's the best choice.
- *Eat Wheat!* **Science:** Yes and no. Skimming the fat off milk creates a lower calorie beverage that is higher in protein and minerals and more difficult to digest. The fats in whole milk, which are not present in skim milk, build and balance the nervous system and act as carriers to deliver the calcium and fat-soluble vitamins A, D3, E, and K directly into the cells. That said, skim milk can be a less *toxic* option... see why below.
- **Dairy Science:** Organic dairy isn't worth the additional cost.
- *Eat Wheat!* **Science:** One of the problems with non-organic dairy is that the chemicals, hormones and toxins in our world are generally fat-soluble. Milk is high up on the food chain, and toxins are therefore passed through the feed into the milk and carried in the fatty portion of the milk. The only way to avoid the overwhelming amounts of antibiotics, growth hormones, and pesticides in milk is to buy organic, where these fat-soluble chemicals are not present.

  If you have to drink non-organic milk, say, at a coffee shop, choose skim milk. Yes, though it is harder to digest, it is virtually devoid of fat and will not carry the hormones, antibiotics and pesticides that whole or low fat milk would.

- **Dairy Science:** Homogenization is a form of milk processing that increases shelf life and improves digestibility.
- *Eat-Wheat!* **Science:** From the Ayurvedic perspective, as well as the perspective of many researchers, the homogenization process renders the fat in milk indigestible. The fat (cream) molecules are squeezed through a very small filter in order to make them homogenous, meaning "the same" as the other molecules in the milk. This homogenous fat is a foreign molecule to the body.[184, 185] This molecule will often pass undigested through weakened small intestinal linings and create foreign sludge, which can stick to walls of the lymph and bloodstream. Some researchers believe this process allows a toxic enzyme called xanthine oxidase to enter into the bloodstream and cause damage to the arterial wall. This arterial free radical damage causes scar tissue to form. Dietary fats can accumulate on the scars and change arterial flow, affecting our health.[186, 187]
- **Dairy-free Science:** Drinking milk causes bloating. Bloating is a sign of lactose intolerance.
- *Eat Wheat!* **Science:** Maybe you're intolerant to the white beverage in the supermarket that is labeled "milk." There are definitely options that are healthier than others when it comes to milk.

Since most milk sold in stores is homogenized, the best choice for milk is organic, vat-pasteurized, non-homogenized milk.

Another non-homogenized milk product is heavy whipping cream. In the production of heavy whipping cream, the cream is skimmed off the milk and never homogenized. Choose organic, because remember that the fat in cream is a carrier for fat-soluble toxins that can find their way into our fat cells or be stored in the brain, and affect our health.[23-27] If organic, non-homogenized, vat-pasteurized milk isn't available, but organic heavy whipping cream is, try adding water to it to make your own "milk."

Traditionally, milk was never consumed in big glasses as it is in the West. Because milk is high in casein (a hard-to-digest protein) and lactose, it was traditionally allowed to separate from the cream. The cream was either churned into butter or eaten in the raw form and saved for cooking in soups. The skim milk was made into cheese or yogurt. The culturing process made the proteins and lactose easier to digest. When milk was called for, cream was simply diluted with water to the desired consistency. In these traditionally prepared foods, cream provided the healthy fats, vitamins A, D, E, and K, and some minerals directly; cheese provided a high-protein, high-mineral product that was easy to digest.

The Magic of Fermentation

Interestingly, only in the West do we regularly drink milk in its natural, or uncultured, form. Traditionally, lacto-fermentation has been generally used to culture milk to preserve it and make it more digestible.

Cheese and yogurts were made to help preserve the dairy through the winter months. As an added bonus, this culturing of milk made it much easier to digest as well. During the fermenting process, Lactobacilli microbes that produce lactic acid proliferate from the souring milk, which preserves the milk while also inhibiting putrefying bacteria.[188] The Lactobacilli bacteria helps to break down—and are also fed by—the milk sugars in dairy. The Lactobacilli are helpful in breaking down the casein in dairy as well.

Casein, a very hard-to-digest protein, is abundant in cow's milk but is not found in high quantities in human mother's milk. The culturing process actually breaks the casein down into easy-to-digest amino acid components. One report states that the proteins in yogurt are digested twice as fast as proteins in unfermented milk.[188] Cheese, kefir, yogurt, and cultured buttermilk are all natural probiotics that support healthy and diverse strains of microbes in the gut. Consider taking small amounts of these cultured, organic, preferably vat-pasteurized dairy products, daily.

Specifically, yogurt is an extremely health-giving food. In India, a meal would not be complete without a dollop of curd or plain, unflavored yogurt to balance a meal. Such ancient wisdom has gained new traction in the medical community.

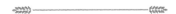

A meta-analysis funded by the National Institutes of Health (NIH) has linked 1 serving of yogurt each day to a 17–18 percent decreased risk of getting type 2 diabetes (T2D).[189] Frank Hu, PhD., a Harvard researcher, pooled the results of 3 large studies that measured the diet and lifestyle of 289,000 health professionals. About 15,000 of them had T2D. While low-fat or full-fat dairy had no measurable effect on T2D risk, yogurt did. 1 serving of yogurt a day decreased the risk of T2D by 17 percent.[189]

Yogurt and yogurt drinks, such as lassi (yogurt and water) and kefir, are considered good for digestion due to their warming properties. This, of course, is especially appreciated in the winter when every bit of warmth helps.

 Tip: Be wary of added sugars in commercial yogurt. You are better off buying plain organic yogurt and adding your own fruit or a small amount of organic maple syrup.

- **Dairy-free Science:** Millions of dollars were spent on research dedicated to prove that saturated fats like ghee and butter are bad for the heart.[190]
- ***Eat Wheat!* Science:** You have probably heard by now that grass-fed is better than grain-fed when it comes to your meat or dairy products. Well, the differences might amaze you!

   Cows grazing grass pastures with no supplemental feed had a whopping 500 percent more conjugated linoleic acid (CLA) in milk fat than cows fed typical grain diets.[191]

   When ghee is organic from grass-fed and pasture-raised cows, it is one of the highest sources of CLA on the planet. CLA has numerous health benefits including boosting immunity, supporting healthy liver function, encouraging bone mass, glucose metabolism, optimal weight, cardiovascular health and antioxidant activity.[192]

Perhaps CLA's most well-documented benefit is its ability to help the body burn fat and lose weight, something dairy is purported to cause.[192, 193] Numerous studies suggest that the ingestion of CLA, short-term or long-term (1 year), significantly reduces the body's fat mass index.[191-193]

Ghee: A Saturated Fat with an Incredible Resume

Ghee is one of the crown jewels of Ayurvedic medicine. It is a delicate, aromatic saturated fat that is solid at room temperature and melts into a liquid as it warms. Ghee is made by boiling off the milk solids (casein, whey, and lactose) from unsalted butter, leaving a very unique blend of heart-healthy fatty acids.

Worried about saturated fat? As it turns out, much of the science telling us for the past 30 years that saturated fats were bad for us was flawed. We now know cholesterol is good for us in the general "total cholesterol" sense. It is the size of both the good (HDL) and bad (LDL) particles along with the amount of triglycerides that determines cardiovascular risk. Study after study, as seen in a scientific meta-analysis, has now negated any association between healthy saturated fats, such as ghee, and cardiovascular issues.[194]

Ghee is the world's best cooking oil! With one of the highest flash points (485°F) of any cooking oil, there are no free radicals or oxidized molecules produced from high-temperature cooking with ghee.

While we think of ghee as a food, according to Ayurveda it was a powerful medicine. Ghee is also loaded with heart, brain, and skin-healthy omega-3 and omega-9 essential fatty acids, along with all the fat-soluble vitamins A, D, E and K, minerals, and at least 9 phenolic antioxidants that support our health and help to prevent disease.[195]

Ghee is also used to detoxify fat-soluble toxins by using a "lipophilic-mediated" detoxification procedure wherein ghee, as a good fat, is ingested to pull (detox) or chelate bad fats or fat-soluble toxins from the body.

Note: In Chapter 12, I have included a 4-day Short Home Cleanse with ghee that incorporates the evidence-based lipophilic-mediated detox practice that has been used for thousands of years.

Butter is Back!

Butter got its name from a fatty acid called butyric acid, and ghee, which is concentrated butter, is the highest known food source of butyric acid on the planet. Butyric acid is the primary fuel for the cells of the colon. It also boosts immunity, feeds the good microbes, and much more.[196]

As it turns out, there are certain microbes in the intestinal tract that are dependent on the carbohydrates and fiber from wheat and other glutenous grains that are genetically wired to make their own butyric acid—no wonder the body loves ghee so much![85] Our daily bread and butter never tasted so good.

Scientists have discovered one of the microbes that actually produces butyric acid in the gut. This microbe, *Clostridium butyricum*, has been used in Asia as a probiotic since the 1940s. It lives naturally in the small and large intestines of healthy folks. Those with compromised digestion were found to have less butyric acid production in the gut.[197] For optimal health, it is important to increase our intake of healthy fats like ghee.

Some of the Benefits of Butyric Acid:[196]
- Helps digestion and maintains the integrity of the gastrointestinal mucosa
- Blocks the growth of bad bacteria in the gut
- Interferes with the growth of highly toxic bacteria
- Helps the growth of beneficial bacteria like Bifidobacterium
- Helps bowel function and regulates abnormal bowel movements
- Helps adjust the water and electrolyte concentration in the intestinal tract

According to one study, the highest sources of Clostridium butyricum are potato skins, yogurt and cream.[198] Think of ghee as basically the fatty acids of cream with all the milk solids boiled off. In another study, the short-chain fatty acid (butyric acid) found in ghee was found to support the health of the intestinal mucosa and normal bowel function in inflammatory bowel conditions.[196] Another very comprehensive study found that butyric acid production in the gut delivers a host of remarkable benefits that extend far beyond the gut:[199]

- Increases insulin sensitivity
- Supports healthy levels of both good and bad cholesterol
- Increases energy production and efficiency of energy utilization
- Reduction in fatty tissue
- Reduction in hunger levels
- Increases thermogenesis in the body

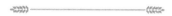

If you are concerned that you may be lactose-intolerant or have difficulty digesting dairy, take the quiz below!

Take the Dairy Quiz

1. **Take organic heavy whipping cream, dilute it with some water, and drink this in place of milk.** If you have issues with the heavy whipping cream, you likely have an issue with fat metabolism and perhaps bile congestion in the liver and/or gallbladder. See Chapter 5 to learn more about your gallbladder's connection to digesting wheat and dairy. The cream is 100 percent fat and has no lactose or casein, which is milk's hard-to-digest protein, so if you have issues here, you may not be lactose intolerant.

2. **Drink skim milk.** If you have issues with skim milk—which has zero fat but does have lactose and casein—then you may be lactose intolerant or you may have a weak digestive fire, meaning decreased production of stomach hydrochloric acid (HCl).

A strong stomach acid is required to break down the casein in dairy, which many folks don't have. Thus, a lack of HCl production in the stomach may be responsible for dairy intolerances.

3. **Eat cheese.** Lactose converts to lactic acid when the dairy is made into cheese, so if you can tolerate cheese, your problem is likely not lactose intolerance. It must be dairy's other culprits—fat or casein, but casein is greatly reduced in cheese, making fat or gallbladder health the concern.

4. **Try whey cheese.** If you cannot tolerate any of the above, try a whey cheese. While there are not many out there (casein is used to make 98 percent of cheeses), whey is a much easier protein to digest. Remember, mother's milk is primarily whey protein, so it is a protein humans know how to digest. Authentic Italian ricotta and Norwegian Gjetost, Prim-ost and Mysost are whey cheeses. To find them, you may need to go to a specialty food store or the European section of your grocery store.

According to Richard Grand, MD, of Harvard Medical School, the bacteria in the gut can learn to grow new lactose-loving bacteria even if you are lactose intolerant.[200] If you feel you are lactose intolerant, try following the plan below.

How to Support Your Gut Microbes in Digesting Lactose Again

1. Start by consuming 1 tablespoon of milk per day and build up to 1 glass per day over a 6-week period of time.

2. It is best to use non-homogenized, vat-pasteurized, organic milk, which is much easier to digest, as it is a non-processed product. Look for Kalona milk or similar vat-pasteurized, non-homogenized, grass-fed, organic dairy products, now sold in natural food stores.

3. This gradual reintroduction of lactose into the diet will allow the gut bacteria to adapt and eventually the gut bacteria will be able to digest lactose without any problem.[200, 201]

Looking Ahead

The issue is not to banish wheat and dairy from your diet because they cause you sensitivity-related symptoms; the deeper issue here is that your digestion is compromised and weak, and that's why you're having trouble digesting these foods.

In Chapter 4, I will dig in and illustrate the importance of the lymph and how it relates to the symptoms we experience when we eat hard-to-digest foods like wheat and dairy.

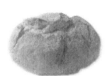

Chapter 4

IT IS NOT THE
GRAIN, IT IS THE
LYMPHATIC DRAINS

M ary[2] came to me complaining of constant migraine headaches, severe sinus pressure, bouts of anxiety and depression, ringing and pain in the ears, rashes all over her body, allergies and achy flu-like joint aches throughout her body. Mary also had a history of severe lifelong digestive issues that oscillated back and forth between constipation and diarrhea.

To help alleviate her symptoms, Mary began by switching to a gluten-free diet, which helped for about a month. She then tried eliminating both gluten *and* dairy from her diet, which helped her for another month or so. Mary then eliminated greasy, fried food on top of her gluten-free and dairy-free diet, which helped as well. However, over time, the symptoms returned. Mary noticed an improvement in how she felt, but all of her symptoms were still not alleviated.

When she started to notice that heavier foods like meat would sit like a rock in her stomach, she switched to being vegetarian. This helped, but her digestive distress persisted. She switched to a vegan diet, and then eventually began eating

---

2   All names of patients have been changed throughout this book to protect their privacy, and all patients have given permission to share the story of their health journey in this book.

an exclusively raw food vegan diet, in search of the perfect diet that she could digest well and that would help her symptoms.

The lighter the foods, the easier she found them to digest, and the better she felt *for a time*. Mary continued to eliminate foods from her diet to feel better, but in the end, this methodology was targeting the symptoms yet ignoring the underlying root of the issue: Weak digestion and the inability to digest hard-to-digest foods.

The symptoms that result when we lose the ability to digest these foods are exactly what Mary was experiencing. When hard-to-digest proteins and fats make their way undigested into the intestines, they will act as intestinal irritants and ooze their way into the lymphatics around the gut, congesting the body's drainage system. The infamous symptoms associated with wheat and dairy sensitivities can be tracked back to congested lymph.

Eliminating more and more foods from the "ok-to-eat" list rarely solves the problem. The goal is to address the root cause of this problem by rebooting the digestive strength so the gluten and casein are being fully digested, and then decongest the clogged lymphatic system responsible for the symptoms of her "food sensitivities."

Let's Talk About Lymph

Hippocrates (460–377 BC) first described the body's lymphatic vessel as "white blood" and coined the term "chyle" from the Greek "chylos," meaning "juice." Chyle is a milky-like fluid consisting of emulsified fats and free fatty acids, collectively called "lymph," which is formed in the digestive system and taken up by the specialized lymph vessels known as lacteals.[16] Proteins and fats are pulled through these intestinal lacteals and routed through over 500 lymph nodes where they are purified by an army of white blood cells. From here, they flow to the heart where they re-enter the circulatory system and end up as cellular nutrition or in the liver where they are ultimately processed.

According to Ayurveda, lymphatic congestion is linked to symptoms including depression, brain fog, migraine headaches, sinus pressure, chronic skin rashes, respiratory and skin allergies, joint pain and a host of digestive imbalances such as gas and bloating.

Additional Symptoms of Lymph Congestion
- Rings get tight on fingers
- Soreness and/or stiffness in the morning
- Feeling tired
- Puffy eyes
- Holding on to water or swelling
- Itchy skin
- Weight gain and extra belly fat
- Swollen glands
- Low immunity
- Breast swelling or soreness with each cycle
- Dry skin
- Mild rash or acne
- Hypersensitivity
- Mild headaches
- Occasional constipation, diarrhea, and/or mucus in the stool

As illustrated in the case study above, Mary lost the ability to digest certain foods, in particular, proteins and hard-to-digest fats. In the intestinal tract, the lymphatic system starts within a series of villi which are tiny finger-like projections that absorb nutrients. Inside the villi, lymphatic lacteals absorb proteins and fats from the intestinal tract into the body's lymphatic system. Particles that are too large to be absorbed into the blood, like numerous fat-soluble toxins and undigested proteins (gluten) can also enter the lymphatic system here.[202] The lymphatic system is the largest circulatory system of the body and although we would all be dead in 24 hours without it, Western science has only just begun to investigate the body's lymph mechanisms.[16, 203]

How the Lymphatic System Works

Ayurvedic medicine, in contrast to Western medicine, has had much to say about the lymph for thousands of years. In fact, the lymphatic system is the very first system of the body that is both evaluated and treated in Ayurveda.

New research in the lymphatic system's multiple roles is confirming what Ayurveda described as "rasa" (which also means juice or lymph), many thousands of years ago. The ancient theory that lymphatic congestion could be a cause of multiple health concerns is now beginning to be an accepted field for scientific investigation.

In general, think of the lymphatic system as the drains in the body. If the drains are clogged, toxins will build up in different areas of the body, causing a variety of lymphatic congestive symptoms such as the sinus pressure, migraine headaches, pain, and hypersensitivity reactions like allergies that Mary experienced.

The proteins found in foods such as wheat, gluten, dairy, casein, soy, nuts, seeds, corn, fish, meat, and other proteins should, in ideal digestion, be properly and efficiently broken down in the upper digestive system. The upper digestive system includes the coordinated effort of the stomach producing acids, the pancreas and duodenum producing digestive enzymes, the liver and gallbladder producing bile, and a host of microbes that digest hard-to-digest proteins and fats found in these foods.

Beneficial intestinal bacteria will digest or disallow the undigested gluten proteins from penetrating the intestinal wall.[72]

When gluten is not completely broken down in the upper digestion, or the intestinal flora is imbalanced, gluten can find its way into the small and large intestines, where the lymph channels can pick them up and take them into the lymphatic system. While 70–80 percent of the body's immune system is found there, the lymph can become overwhelmed by a lifetime of processed foods and poor digestion.[11, 204, 205]

Once the intestinal wall becomes inflamed or irritated, the intestinal lymphatic system can be exposed to a variety of environmental toxins such as xenobiotics or undigested proteins such as the gliadins from poorly digested wheat that are too large to enter into the blood.[202, 206]

The intestinal lymphatics are where the body's initial immune T-cell response against undigested glutens takes place in an attempt to purify them. Typically, when the intestinal wall is healthy, undigested proteins and toxins would be taken into the bloodstream and escorted to the liver where they would be detoxified.[207]

Unfortunately, once these toxins or gluten enter a congested lymphatic system, there is limited detoxification there and the allergic, chemically sensitive or gluten sensitive symptoms can quickly become a problem. In general, the lymphatic system is better equipped to fight bacteria and viruses than to break down toxins, which happens in the liver, or digest proteins, which happens in the stomach and small intestine.

That said, the lymphatic system seems to have a back-up plan for gluten and other undigested proteins that happen to enter the lymph as a result of a broken down intestinal system. There is a naturally-occurring digestive enzyme called dipeptidyl peptidase IV (DPP-IV) which is typically found in the duodenum, that has also been found in the lymph surrounding the small intestine. DPP-IV has been shown to break down gluten and gliadin, which suggests that some digesting of gluten will take place in the lymph as well as the small intestine. If the small intestine however becomes inflamed, the lymph will congest and inflame as well, compromising lymph flow and the breakdown of gluten both in the duodenum and the lymph.[208, 209]

Lymph and Brain Fog

Western medicine now agrees with Ayurveda that there are lymphatic channels all over the body. However, until recently, Western medicine concluded that the brain and the nervous system were completely devoid of lymphatic channels!

A recent groundbreaking study performed at the University of Virginia School of Medicine, which I discussed earlier in this book, has discovered lymphatic channels called glymphatics that literally drain the brain and central nervous system (CNS) of toxins and beta-amyloid plaque.

Thousands of years ago, Ayurveda had described lymphatic channels that drain the sagittal sinus of the brain and mirror the pattern of a Mohawk haircut. This is exactly where modern researchers found the lymphatic vessels that drain the brain of toxins and other waste material![5] Congestion of these glymphatics are linked to poor cognitive function, brain inflammation, autoimmune conditions, depression, brain fog and Alzheimer's disease.[5, 210]

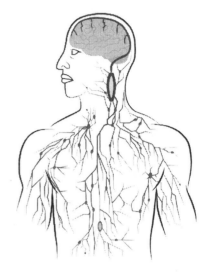

While you sleep, particularly if you sleep on your side, it takes about 6–8 hours for the brain to completely drain its toxins that may have accumulated throughout the day. On average, the brain drains about 3 pounds of these toxins each year.[211]

Inflammation anywhere in the body can affect the circulation of the blood and lymph. New research suggests that the brain and CNS glymphatic vessels can also be congested as a result of inflammation and infection. Infections, which are fought in the lymphatic system along with inflammation, have been linked to depression and other mood-related disorders. This groundbreaking research suggests that many mental health concerns may not actually be psychological, but instead physiological.[8, 212]

The glymphatic vessels regulate the circulation of mood-balancing neurotransmitters such as GABA in the brain. Glymphatic congestion can be linked to brain fog, cognitive concerns, anxiety and depression—all of which are associated with wheat and dairy allergies.

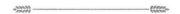

The new science is linking problems of the mind to problems of the body, particularly in the digestion and lymph.[213]

Let's Further Explore Lymphatic Congestion

If the skin of the intestinal tract breaks down due to mental, physical, or emotional stress, poor diet, or unhealthy lifestyle choices, the villi and lacteals of the intestinal tract will also break down. These villi and lacteals are some of the key players for absorbing nutrients, vitamins, minerals, *and* removing toxins.[214, 215] When these are not functioning correctly, undigested foods like proteins and fats can enter into the gut-associated and mesenteric lymphatic tissue that surrounds the large and small intestines.[11-15] These undigested proteins and fats that build up in the lymphatic system can cause hypersensitivity reactions or allergic reactions throughout the lymphatic system.

Many studies show that when the lymphatic tissue becomes congested with toxins or hard-to-digest proteins and fats, the lymphatic system can overflow into the fat layers around the gut and predispose the body to various forms of obesity and health concerns.

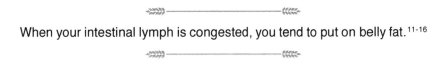

When your intestinal lymph is congested, you tend to put on belly fat.[11-16]

Furthermore, researchers have also found that congested lymph, full of toxins, can move into the body's fat cells and intercellular spaces, causing toxicity that has been linked to the production and metastasis of tumors.[16-19] This all starts in the digestive system.

Thus, a decongested lymphatic system is important to ward off not only food allergy-related symptoms like bloating, gas, and brain fog from foods like wheat and dairy, but also to help protect us from more serious imbalances. This is just the beginning of your new understanding of the lymph.

Got Cellulite?

When the intestinal lymphatic tissue becomes congested, not only will the belly swell and become bloated, gassy, and carry extra weight, the lymphatic system will also be unable to efficiently carry intercellular fluid waste from every cell of the body back upwards towards the heart for proper processing.[16] Lymph and cellular waste products from your feet, legs, thighs, pass through the abdominal lymph vessels around the belly back to the heart en route to the liver.

If that lymphatic tissue is congested, the fluid waste can back up into the lymph around your hips and thighs, predisposing the body to levels of microcirculation, lymphatic congestion, and manifest as varicose veins or cellulite. Lymph drainage techniques have been scientifically found to help reduce cellulite.[216, 217]

As the lymphatic system is draining waste back to the heart via muscular contractions rather than the pumping of the heart, there is a tendency for the hands, feet, legs and thighs to be areas vulnerable to lymphatic congestion. This can manifest in a number of concerns from skin rashes to arthritic pain to weight gain and swelling in those areas.

Why Exercise is Important for a Healthy Lymphatic System

The lymphatic system is stimulated by exercise, movement and muscular contractions. Inside every muscle is a lymphatic vessel that is pumping waste back to the heart with every muscular contraction. This is also why there can be early morning stiffness when you get out of bed. This is a classic sign of lymphatic congestion, because at night, when you're not moving or walking, the lymph has a tendency to pool, resulting in morning stiffness.

As a result, it can take a little while to get the lymph pumping again and for your body to feel less puffy and stiff. The benefits of exercise and breathing are incredibly important for healthy lymphatic flow and eradicating the symptoms of gluten sensitivity. Chapter 13 is dedicated to a lymph-focused exercise called The *Eat Wheat* Workout.

Journey through the Lymph

When certain unwanted proteins and fats find their way through the intestinal wall into the lymphatic tissue, there are a series of lymph nodes full of immune responders designed to take care of them.[218] In small amounts, the body is well equipped to process these undigested proteins and fats. In large amounts, undigested glutens can overwhelm the lymph, leading to food and environmental sensitivities.

Once the toxins and undigested proteins enter into the intestinal lymphatic tissue, they move through different aspects of the lymphatic system. One of the main channels is called the skin-associated lymphatic tissue (SALT).[219]

Think of your skin when you get a mosquito bite. The skin gets red, and the skin-associated lymphatic tissue, which carries an army of white blood cells right beneath your skin, is ready to pounce on any bacteria or virus that might be carried by the mosquito bite.

When the lymphatic system is working well, the immune system attacks the invader and all is taken care of. Wherever there is skin on the body, there is a lymphatic army waiting on the other side just beneath the skin.[218] In the intestinal tract, *which is also made of skin,* the gut-associated lymphatic tissue (GALT), which is the largest concentration of lymph in the body outside the intestinal wall, stands ready to pounce and protect the body from anything that is undesirable trying to cross over the intestinal wall.[220]

Gluten and dairy intolerances are a result of a long-term overwhelming breakdown of digestive strength. As digestive power decreases, these hard-to-digest proteins and fats are allowed to enter into the lymph and cause a host of lymphatic-related symptoms.

Exit-Ramp through the Skin

If the skin-associated lymph is congested or the lymphatic system is stuck in traffic, then the immune system will also become stuck in traffic, and the skin may end up becoming an exit ramp for impurities to move out of the body in the form of skin rashes, hives, eczema, acne or other types of skin concerns. The skin can also swell and inflame when the lymphatic system is congested. Rings might get tight on fingers, the eye area may get puffy, ankles might swell, and the whole body can begin to hold onto more fluid and swell. These are all classic lymphatic-related symptoms.

Exit-Ramp through the Respiratory System

Another important lymphatic pathway is the respiratory-associated lymphatic tissue, otherwise known as the mucus-associated lymphatic tissue (MALT) or larynx-associated lymphatic tissue (LALT). These are the lymphatic tracts that drain the respiratory skin.[221]

Once again, on the outside of the respiratory tract, there is an army of lymphatic immune help ready to pounce on any irritants that pass through the respiratory skin. If the cilia of the respiratory tract become either too dry or too mucus-filled, just like the tale of the three little bears, with the conditions needing to be "just right," the cilia will not be able to process waste or toxins through the respiratory tract efficiently, which can cause a hypersensitivity reaction.

This, in turn, can cause the lymphatic system waiting beneath the cilia to once again congest, causing symptoms such as sore throats, swollen glands and headaches. Once the toxins from undigested proteins and fat move from the intestinal lymph, the entire lymphatic system can become congested, compounding the problem and making the body more vulnerable to immune-related issues.

In the respiratory tract, this can result in hypersensitivity reactions to pollens and pollutants. It can cause chemical sensitivities and allergies, as well as predispose the body to the proliferation of undesirable bacteria and viruses that can cause a cold, flu, or other types of infection.

Congestion in the respiratory lymph can also cause a host of lymphatic-related symptoms including allergies, asthma, ear aches and even migraines, acne, skin rashes and psoriasis on the head and neck, ringing of the ears, brain fog, and mood-related issues like anxiety and depression. Thyroid concerns can be related to lymph congestion, according to Ayurveda, since the thyroid is drained by cervical lymph. If the lymph drainage is congested, the thyroid, which is located in the neck, cannot communicate well with the higher centers, such as the brain, and the lower centers, such as the rest of the body.

Over time, the thyroid can become congested and begin to turn on itself, as the immune system all too often responds overzealously to toxins in the lymph-associated thyroidal tissue, predisposing the body to an autoimmune reaction such as Hashimoto's disease. Congested lymph can also cause the immune system to either become weak, compromised, or over-reactive, which can trigger autoimmune reactions elsewhere in the body.[5]

Lymph and the Reproductive System

Prior to menstruation and right after ovulation, there is an internal detoxification that takes place through lymphatic vessels that drain the reproductive system.10 Due to the congestion of the lymph, women can experience PMS symptoms like bloating, breast swelling and tenderness, weight gain, acne and moodiness, as the body tries to move waste into an already congested lymphatic system.

If the lymphatic system is congested as a result of years of digestive imbalances, toxins can also build up in the reproductive system, causing a host of reproductive health concerns that are often treated as hormonal imbalances. By decongesting the lymphatic system, which I will discuss in Part II, many of the symptoms prior to menstruation can lessen or disappear entirely. It is interesting that we now have a link between lymphatic congestion and mood-related concerns; that which physically congests us can correlate with our emotional congestion.

In A Nutshell

1. The lymphatic system starts inside the intestinal tract of your digestive system. If the lymph is clogged or congested, digestion will be off, and numerous health concerns can arise. Because the lymph system is systemic, the symptoms of gluten sensitivity can manifest anywhere in the body. Most commonly the symptoms of food intolerance manifest where the lymph is most predominant, e.g., the brain, nervous system, lungs, skin and the entire digestive system.

2. The upper digestive system, which is responsible for breaking down these foods, is often imbalanced and may make it impossible for the intestinal skin and the lacteals of the lymphatic system to do their job properly, leaking toxins, undigested gluten and casein into the lymph.

3. In addition, problems arise when these foods are overeaten and consumed out of season on a regular basis.

4. Modern processing causes dairy and wheat, in particular, to become lymph-congesting and difficult to digest.

5. Stress directly impacts the health and function of the intestinal skin and its microbes,[222] which do the heavy lifting for almost every function of the body.[66] When stress is chronic, it is in part responsible for the breakdown of the intestinal skin and aspects of the digestive process and the congestion of the lymphatic system. (Read more on this in Chapter 9, 13 and 14.)

The good news is that all of these issues are easily fixed and easily brought back into balance allowing most of my patients to enjoy wheat and dairy once again while protecting themselves against more serious health concerns.

Looking Ahead

Remember how Mary naturally chose a diet that was easier to digest, though taking a trip down the increasingly restrictive dietary lane? While these dietary restrictions gave her symptomatic relief, it did not actually solve the root of her problem—her weak digestive strength. In Part II of this book, we will dig into how I helped balance Mary's health issues, which were related to lymphatic congestion and hard-to-digest foods.

Chapter 5 will explore how the upper digestion is letting hard-to-digest proteins like wheat and dairy go undigested in the first place.

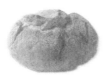

THE GREAT
DIGESTIVE
BREAKDOWN

The Evolution of Digesting Gluten

F ully understanding how the human body digests gluten is very much a scientific work in progress. There is emerging science that is helping us understand why the body has a difficult time fully breaking down gluten. After millions of years of gluten-digesting evolution, the body knows exactly what it is doing when it comes to gluten, and contrary to what many believe, it is not a poison after all.

The latest science is suggesting that some of the gluten consumed may never have been intended to be fully digested. Many of the undigested gluten proteins are escorted into the large intestine, where they dramatically increase the numbers of beneficial gut bacteria. In one study, a gluten-rich diet increased certain enzymes in the large intestine called glutenases, which fully break down the gliadins found in gluten. Here in the large intestine, the gluten acted as a fuel supply for good gut microbes. These microbes were found to boost the production of beneficial short chain fatty acids (SCFA) like the butyric acid that I discussed in Chapter 3. The more gluten in the diet, the more glutanase activity and SCFA production they found. Extra gluten was found excreted in the stools.[223]

This study concluded that gluten digestion may have evolved to only be partially broken down in the small intestine in healthy people, in order to supply the large intestine with important food for the gut microbes. It seems that a major underlying factor causing wheat, dairy and food sensitivities is linked to the health of the upper digestion.[223]

When the lining of the small intestine is damaged, these undigested proteins can act as intestinal irritants and find their way into the lymphatic system where they are linked to numerous immune and health concerns. Protecting the integrity of the upper digestion and the intestinal skin is not a new concept. It has been the premise of Ayurveda for thousands of years, and a major focus of this book.

While some of the gluten ingested is earmarked to enter the large intestine, there are also numerous gluten-digesting enzymes and bacteria in the upper digestive system, suggesting that at least in part, gluten was a nutritional source to be broken down and absorbed through the small intestine as well.

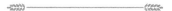

According to a new study, the body starts digesting all of the very hard-to-digest gluten proteins as soon as we put it in our mouths. A multitude of gluten- and gliadin-degrading enzymes were found in normal human saliva that were manufactured by a variety of naturally-occurring oral bacteria.

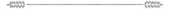

The saliva, which is loaded with both the gluten-digesting enzymes and oral bacteria, is produced and swallowed in quantities of up to a liter a day. The oral bacteria and enzymes that are swallowed stay active in a wide pH range, suggesting that this gluten-digesting activity extends into the esophagus and small intestine.[224]

Not to mention the numerous microbes that can break down gluten, there are also naturally-occurring digestive enzymes in both the pancreas and duodenal mucosa, such as Dipeptidyl peptidase IV (DPP-IV) that break down the gliadins found in gluten and the casein found in dairy. Most active in the brush border of the duodenum, DPP-IV has been shown to completely break down proline-containing epitope of gliadin, the primary allergenic protein in gluten. DPP-IV has also been shown to markedly enhance the gluten- and casein-degrading capacity of other protein-digesting enzymes. This is the same enzyme that I discussed in Chapter 4, that can help break down undigested proteins like gluten and casein in the lymphatic systm.[208, 209]

All of these digestive enzymes, along with the gluten-digesting bacteria and probiotics I introduced in Chapter 1, depend on a balanced digestive system and the healthy lining of the stomach, small and large intestinal skin. This can be repaired, but first, let's discuss how we got into this mess in the first place.

The Beginning of the End

For the past forty-plus years, Americans ate fewer eggs and other animal products because the government concluded cholesterol and fat were bad for us. High cholesterol foods ended up on the government's nutrient concern list[28] based on a misinterpreted study on rabbits done in the early 1900s.[225]

As a result of this verdict against cholesterol, foods were manufactured without it. Animal fats like butter were considered unhealthy, eggs were taboo, fatty foods were replaced with non-fat foods and, overnight, America found itself on a pervasively low-fat, low-cholesterol, carbohydrate-heavy diet. The problem, unfortunately, was that this low-fat diet did not reduce cholesterol levels, nor did it reduce cardiovascular risk. In fact, this low-cholesterol diet took away the important fuel supply from the body that humans have been eating for thousands of years—saturated fat.

Our ancient hunter-gatherer ancestors dug up roots and gathered grains, greens, berries, and seeds, as well as hunted. And while our early ancestors were likely more prolific gatherers than hunters, there is no doubt that hunting was an extremely important part of our evolution as humans. Many researchers believe that our brain literally tripled in size with the ingestion of more saturated animal fats.[226]

In 1961, when these saturated fats were put on the government's nutrient concern list and taken out of our diet for the very first time in thousands upon thousands of years,[28] they were replaced by a different fuel supply. Wheat and corn replaced fat as the nation's fuel supply, and in short order, America was fueled by sugar.[65]

Wheat and corn quickly became the new "it" foods in America.[28, 65] They had obvious appeal in certain ways. They were cheap to grow and easily processed into foods that would sit on the shelves for months, as well as be easily processed into sugars like high-fructose corn syrup. Sugar packs a short burst of energy. It is fuel that helps you run away from a bear, get up a tree and save your life. However, sugar is not a sustaining fuel; it's more of a rollercoaster ride. We burn it fast ("the sugar high"), and our blood sugar crashes after it's all burned up.

Fats, on the other hand, are the preferred source of fuel for humans, as they provide long-lasting, stable, calm, non-emergency, sleep-through-the-night, handle-stress, no-anxiety fuel.

As a result of this switch to simple carbohydrates to replace fat, as a culture, we have lost our ability to stay calm and burn fat as a stable source of fuel. Consider this: More than a third of Americans are obese. We find ourselves with a global anxiety and depression problem. Kids cannot sit still in class, people cannot sleep through the night, and people cannot eat enough food to become satisfied. All of these can be linked to a diet high in sugar and low in good fat.

The unintended result of this low-cholesterol, high-sugar diet has set America up for an epidemic of blood sugar-related problems.[227, 228] This problem has been blamed on gluten, but as we saw in Chapters 1 and 2, there is plenty of science to the contrary. Gluten-free foods are poised to take the pre-diabetic epidemic to an even more dangerous height. Most of the gluten-free foods are highly processed, hard to find completely organic and rendered with a higher glycemic index than unprocessed whole wheat breads.[229, 230] Intestinal permeability and leaky gut has been linked to the processed foods in our diet, so please beware that it is likely the processed nature of our diet in the U.S.—which is much more processed than the food supply in Europe[231]—that is behind so many food sensitivities and food intolerances.[232]

Thankfully, in 2014, the governmental committee that develops the country's dietary guidelines lifted their low-fat diet recommendation. In 2015, longstanding caps on dietary cholesterol were removed, stating there was "no appreciable relationship" between blood cholesterol and dietary cholesterol. The low-fat, no cholesterol era has finally ended![28]

Who Needs a Gallbladder?

Without adequate cholesterol and fat in the diet, the gallbladder can become sluggish, as it requires a certain amount of fat to exercise itself and stay functional. In one study, it was suggested that the leading cause of gallbladder disease is, in fact, a highly touted low-fat diet.[233] The U.S. has been on a poor-quality-fat diet for almost 50 years, and slowly we have seen a steady rise in gallbladder issues,[234] which are directly linked to both a weak lower and upper digestion.

It is interesting to note that we have a record number of gallbladder surgeries in America. Most people don't even have to change their diet after they have their gallbladder removed, suggesting that maybe we don't really need the gallbladder anymore. Perhaps we've actually evolved away from needing the little storage sac of bile called the gallbladder.

I would like you to reconsider any notion you may have that the gallbladder is unimportant or expendable. The reality is that the gallbladder holds a sack of bile that is 15 times the concentration of the bile produced from the liver.[203, 235]

Considering our ancient ancestors, it might be logical to deduce that this kind of bile production was used to digest, perhaps, the brains and the intestines of a woolly mammoth. Eating such large amounts of fat in one sitting followed by periods of no fat tends to force the gallbladder to contract in a major way, decongesting any possible bile and liver congestion.

Today, we have just the opposite problem. We find ourselves with either inadequate amounts of good fats or an abundance of indigestible processed fats in order to produce an adequate amount of bile. As a result, the bile that is reabsorbed from the intestines to the liver is reused on average up to 17 times before it is discarded. It's like washing our dishes in the same dirty dishwater 17 times in a row![203]

The reason why the bile would be reused so often was likely a survival tool in times of famine. When fats were scarce, humans had the ability to reuse bile again and again until hunters brought a new supply of fatty meat. As a result, today we have 94 percent of our bile—with all the toxins in tow—being reabsorbed back to the liver,[203] circulating toxins back into the bloodstream where they oxidize our good cholesterol and are potentially being stored in our fat cells and even our brains.[23-27]

It is this lack of bile flow and bile production that is a major contributor of the slow and steady shutting down of the production of stomach acid. The lack of stomach acid and its coordination with the liver, gallbladder, pancreas and duodenum all contribute to our inability to digest hard-to-digest foods like wheat and dairy.

Lack of bile flow is also responsible for the consistency of the stools. It is the bile that regulates the stool. Plain and simple: No bile, no poop. No bile, no stomach acid. Thus, one can experience poor and painful digestion of wheat, dairy, and fatty foods.

Note: Before you start increasing the fats in your diet, you must first stop eating sugar, processed foods and reboot the function of the gallbladder. More on this in Part II.

Let's take a journey through one person's digestive system to better understand exactly how it can weaken and break down, and what can be done to resolve these issues and heal from the inside out. This is the story of Daniel,[3] a patient who came to see me in 2014.

Daniel's Story

Daniel came to see me complaining of anxiety, chest pain, and shortness of breath. When a patient shares symptoms like these, I immediately recommend

---

3   All names of patients have been changed throughout this book to protect their privacy, and all patients have given permission to share the story of their health journey in this book.

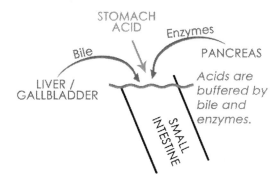

Getting Acquainted with Your Digestive Anatomy

they get checked out by a cardiologist, and then I do my best to dig into the cause of the problem.

Daniel had a history of constipation as a child, which had become chronic, and was now experiencing alternating bouts of constipation, diarrhea, and mucus in the stool. He also complained about heartburn, gas and bloating, and years of indigestion.

He told me he had stopped eating fatty or fried food and any heavy or rich food, for that matter years ago, because it would make his heartburn worse. He would either end up with a feeling of nausea or the food would just sit there like a rock.

In an attempt to solve his digestive issues, he told me he had experimented with taking foods out of his diet. First, he removed most fatty foods, then wheat and dairy. Like Mary, he reported feeling somewhat better each time he took another food group out of his diet. While each food elimination worked for a time, the symptoms kept returning.

Daniel was like so many of my patients. He experienced an initial benefit in removing wheat and dairy, but the benefit didn't last. The symptoms return even without these foods. This is not to say that wheat and dairy will not exacerbate such symptoms, they often do, which is why so many people understandably choose to avoid these foods. But once again, this elimination approach to food sensitivities treats the effect, the symptoms, when we need to be treating the cause in order to stay healthy and prevent more serious health concerns in the future.

After years of adjusting his diet and eliminating more and more foods, Daniel began to experience bouts of anxiety, chest pain, and shortness of breath, which is when he came to see me. What is interesting about all of Daniel's symptoms is that they're all linked to an underlying digestive imbalance. The body never does anything without a good reason. Each symptom is a logical expression of the body trying to deal with a history of constipation and resultant lymph congestion. Each symptom represents the body trying to move impurities out through alternative detoxification pathways other than its main, clogged waste removal channels.

Digestion 101

In Daniel's case, the history of constipation caused chronic dryness in the intestinal mucous membranes. The intestinal skin, like the respiratory skin, cannot be too dry or too wet with mucus.[236] The conditions have to be just right for the microbes that support optimal health to proliferate and for the neurotransmitters manufactured in the gut to stabilize mood and support the nervous system.[237-252]

If the intestinal tract becomes too dry or too wet, the villi and lacteals of the intestinal wall can break down, predisposing the intestinal tract to irritation, damage, and a type of leaky gut syndrome that allows these toxins and hard-to-digest proteins to enter the body's lymphatic system, creating the perfect storm for food intolerances.[236, 253-255]

When the skin of the intestinal tract breaks down and toxins cannot be removed through the congested intestinal lymphatics (where many of the gluten symptoms first manifest), the toxins will eventually be redirected through the enteric cycle back to the liver.

The liver's job is to break down fats and toxins that have been processed through the intestines and lymphatic system, and to gobble them up with bile.

What's Bile and Liver Got to do with it?

Bile is like a Pac-Man inside the liver, gobbling up toxins, fatty acids, environmental pollutants, pesticides, cholesterol, and other fatty impurities. When we ingest fatty foods, for instance, the bile is secreted from the liver and gallbladder into the intestinal tract, where it continues to gobble up more of the same—toxins, fatty acids, environmental pollutants, preservatives, chemicals, parasites, and other undesirable bacteria, just to name a few.[256]

Once the bile gets into the intestinal tract, it attaches itself to fiber in the gut and is escorted to the toilet with all the toxins in tow. This is a wonderfully efficient process of removing waste, as long as we have enough fiber in our diet to get the job done.

Our hunter-gatherer ancestors ate about 100 grams of fiber each day. The average American has 15–20 grams of fiber in their diet each day.[257] So as a result, our ancestors had about 5 times more fiber in their diet than we do, and therefore had at least 5 times the efficiency of fat-soluble waste removal than we do. Bile, which is attached to numerous toxins, will be reabsorbed back into the liver, back into circulation, instead of being eliminated and escorted into the toilet if we have an inadequate amount of fiber in our diet.

Once the liver becomes overwhelmed with detoxification projects, such as dealing with recirculated toxic bile, the liver can become congested and these toxic fats can literally build up in the liver, causing a well-known condition called "fatty liver" while oxidizing or damaging the good healthy cholesterols. Oxidized cholesterol particles are now understood to be the real culprit of the cholesterol-based cardiovascular risk. More importantly, the congestion in the liver can cause a lack of bile production, a lack of bile flow, and a thickening or increased viscosity of the bile itself. Thick, viscous bile can congest the bile ducts and literally turn off the digestive process and the ability to break down wheat and dairy.[258]

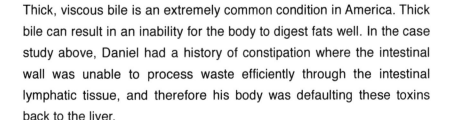

Thick, viscous bile is an extremely common condition in America. Thick bile can result in an inability for the body to digest fats well. In the case study above, Daniel had a history of constipation where the intestinal wall was unable to process waste efficiently through the intestinal lymphatic tissue, and therefore his body was defaulting these toxins back to the liver.

Once Daniel's liver became congested and his bile became thick, he was unable to digest fatty foods. Being able to digest and deliver good fats to the brain, heart, skin and nervous system is critically important. Over time, lack of healthy fat metabolism can cause an inability to keep the nervous system stable and predisposes many people to anxiety and other stress-related concerns, similar to what Daniel was experiencing.[259]

When Daniel did eat some fatty food, and there was insufficient bile to break it down, the stomach chose to hold onto the fats and wait for the bile to be produced. In Daniel's case, the constipation and bile congestion became chronic, leaving Daniel with an inadequate supply of bile to break down fats. As a result, the stomach was holding onto the fats longer than it should've, and Daniel would feel nauseous and heavy. Without adequate bile to digest a fatty meal, the heavy or fatty foods would just sit there like a rock and not digest— sound familiar?

Why Eliminating Foods is Not a Sustainable Solution

Avoiding fatty foods was Daniel's initial solution to this problem, but it didn't last. Here is why:

The bile in the gallbladder and liver not only emulsifies fats, but it also buffers acids such as the hydrochloric acid (HCl) in the stomach. When the stomach is trying to break down hard-to-digest proteins like gluten in wheat and the casein in dairy, it requires a very strong production of stomach acid.

If there is limited bile production in the liver, the stomach will sometimes hold onto the excess acid, as if to wait for the bile to be produced in order to buffer the harsh stomach acids. This is a very common cause for experiencing symptoms of heartburn. According to a recent survey, 44 percent of Americans experience heartburn at least once a month, and about 7 percent or 22 million Americans experience a daily bout of heartburn.[260, 261]

In some cases, the stomach will allow the acids to leave the stomach in an attempt to protect the stomach lining from excess acid. When this happens without adequate bile to buffer those acids, the acids may burn and damage the intestinal wall, causing duodenal ulcers, intestinal irritation, leaky gut, and a detrimental alteration in the intestinal microbiology. Unbuffered acids from the stomach moving into the intestinal tract could cause severe intestinal inflammatory symptoms, which would make the intestinal tract and lymphatic system even more vulnerable and susceptible to being irritated by hard-to-digest or undigested proteins from wheat and dairy.

The stomach will try its best to hold onto the stomach acid for as long as possible, but in time, the excess acid will irritate the stomach lining, setting the body up for chronic gas, bloating, indigestion and bouts of nausea, heartburn and shortness of breath, as seen in Daniel's case. Daniel's history of constipation may have caused congestion of the liver and gallbladder, compromising bile flow, the ability to digest fats and the inability to effectively buffer the stomach's digestive acids.[262]

Intestinal irritation from a lack of bile flow or the passing of unbuffered stomach acids into the intestines can also cause bouts of diarrhea with mucus either lining the stool or mixed into the looser stool, which we saw in Daniel's case history. Mucus production in the stool is common and often caused by excessive stress and worry along with the breakdown of the upper digestive process.

Is it a Hiatal Hernia?

When the stomach is pushing so persistently in an upward direction onto the diaphragm that the stomach literally herniates through the lower esophageal sphincter and the diaphragmatic wall, it's considered a "hiatal hernia." The stomach is designed to hang down off the diaphragm and not push up against it. This kind of chronic upward pushing of the stomach onto the diaphragm is common, and can be the result of poor bile flow and the delayed emptying of the stomach acids and fats as I previously described. Pregnancy can also exacerbate this tendency, as the baby naturally puts upward pressure on the stomach and diaphragm.[263] Normally, after delivery, the stomach returns to its original position, but many women never feel quite the same after they have had their babies, and this may be why.

In the case of a hiatal hernia, for example, the upward pressure took years for the stomach to actually herniate through the lower esophageal sphincter of the diaphragm. Years before the stomach herniates, bouts of chronic heartburn and indigestion could be putting undue pressure on the diaphragm and sometimes even adhering parts of the stomach wall to the underside of the diaphragm. As you might expect, when this happens, neither the stomach nor diaphragm can function well and this area can become very tight and tender. Unfortunately, this is extremely common in my patients with food intolerances. (In Chapter 10, I will share a home exercise called "stomach pulling" to help resolve this problem.)

 Tip: Check for soreness, tightness or pain on the abdomen, just under the ribs or both sides.

As a result of Daniel's long-standing constipation, toxins were reabsorbed back into the liver where his bile ducts became congested, resulting in the holding on to stomach acid and heartburn. Daniel was a tricky case, because not only did we need to free up his stomach and diaphragm, we needed to decongest his bile ducts and bring his elimination back into balance. I will how to do this, step by step, in Part II.

In Daniel's case, the diaphragm itself became unable to fully contract and pull air deeply into the lower lobes of the lungs. This is important because the lower lobes of the lungs are where a predominance of parasympathetic nerve receptors is located. When we breathe deeply into the lower lobes of the lungs, we activate the calming, rest-and-digest parasympathetic nervous system. When we lose access to the lower lobes of the lungs, the tendency is to breathe only into the upper lobes, where there is a predominance of fight-or-flight nerve receptors.[264, 265]

Commonly, this can be the cause of chest pressure and difficulty breathing, as we saw in Daniel's case. In this case, it is also common to experience yourself frequently trying to catch your breath, getting side aches when you run, feeling out of shape, and this can even contribute to asthma, allergies, snoring and sleep apnea. There are also lymph vessels that drain the lungs and respiratory system that, when congested as a result of digestive imbalance, can be linked to a host of congestive respiratory concerns.[266] Yoga and backward stretches that open the chest and stomach area helped Daniel resolve his breathing and chest pressure considerably. I will describe these in Chapter 13.

Dialing down Wheat and Dairy Digestion

Over time, the stomach lining can become irritated, inflamed, and even ulcerated from the HCl build-up that is lingering in the stomach due to poor or congested bile flow. In an attempt to protect itself from the lingering HCl, the stomach can make an executive decision to turn down the stomach fire, decreasing the production of stomach acid to match the lack of production of bile in the liver and gallbladder.

> If there is inadequate production of bile, there will be a lack of production of stomach acid.[262] Without adequate production of stomach acid, hard-to-digest proteins like gluten and dairy will simply not be initially digested and broken down.

Pancreatic Enzymes

In 91 percent of people, the bile duct and the pancreatic duct join together before they enter into the small intestine.[203] If the bile ducts have become congested, as in Daniel's case, and like I commonly see in my practice, the pancreatic ducts will also become congested, blocking pancreatic digestive enzymes from moving into the intestinal tract to support the buffering of stomach acids and the breaking down of hard-to-digest foods.

There is a coordinated effort between the stomach producing the appropriate amount of HCl that triggers the release of bile, which triggers the release of pancreatic enzymes, which triggers release of the duodenal enzymes. All of these are required to create the perfect environment for the intestinal microbiology to proliferate. When both intestinal environment and upper digestion are healthy and the digestive process is coordinated, only then are elements required for a healthy microbiome and the digestion of wheat and dairy in place.

The Skinny on Digestive Supplements

Many of my patients find benefit from taking digestive enzymes. Many naturopaths and medical professionals suggest that, as we age, we simply stop producing digestive acid in the stomach, bile flow in the liver, and pancreatic enzymes from the pancreas. Others find themselves propping up their weak digestion by taking HCl pills, pancreatic enzyme pills, and herbal laxative pills to keep their digestive system moving along.

The reality is that the vast majority of Americans have thick, viscous bile as a result of eating highly processed food over many years. This has not only congested the bile and pancreatic ducts, but has shut down the optimal production of acid in the stomach—all of which are required to detox and digest well. When the bile becomes thick and the bile ducts congested, the pancreatic duct also becomes blocked. Pancreatic digestive enzymes simply cannot get through the congested bile ducts to do their job. As a result, you may reach for digestive enzymes. This may help alleviate the symptoms, but as you can see, once again we are only treating the symptoms and not the cause of the issue, which can set us up for other health issues down the road.

Instead of investing in digestive enzymes or other digestive aids, consider a more efficient and long-term plan to target the root cause—your digestion.

Looking Ahead

Read on to discover how I helped Daniel stimulate bile flow, and strengthen and balance weak digestion in Part II of this book. It is time to take action and reboot your digestion so you can once again—or perhaps for the first time that you can remember—enjoy your bread and butter!

— PART II —
The Fix—Igniting the Digestive Fire within You

"When diet is wrong, medicine is of no use, when diet is correct, medicine is of no need."

——Ayurvedic Proverb

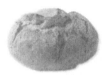

Chapter 6
EAT WHEAT: HOW,
WHEN AND WHAT KIND

B irds fly south, whales migrate, and flowers bloom in a perfect symphony between nature's rhythms and all of its life forms. Life—not to mention our digestion—is tied to these cycles that science calls circadian rhythms.[267]

Is it possible that the most subtle forces in nature can be the most powerful? The microbiome for example, houses trillions of microscopic bacteria that impact every function in the body.[66] Today, scientists are suggesting that the circadian clock, which we cannot see or touch, could revolutionize medicine as we know it.

New science is suggesting that we have become disconnected from these cycles. Our genes, found in every cell of the body, have become unable to hear or respond to the circadian rhythms of nature.[267] This will have an impact on every aspect of our health.

To evaluate your connection to these rhythms and how this affects your digestion and your health, please take this short Circadian Rhythms Quiz to help you understand how easy it is to fall out of sync with the cycles of nature.

Circadian Rhythms Quiz

1. Whenever possible, do you prefer to sleep in after the sunrise?   Yes or No

2. Do you wake up stiff and take a while to get going?   Yes or No

3. Do you work through your lunch or skip lunch so you can leave work early or lose weight?   Yes or No

4. Do you eat the same basic diet, more or less, throughout the year?   Yes or No

5. Do you have trouble getting to sleep or staying asleep?   Yes or No

6. Do you crave snacks, even healthy ones, throughout the day?   Yes or No

7. Do you regularly eat dinner after 7 p.m.?   Yes or No

8. Do you get tired in the afternoon around 3–4 o'clock?   Yes or No

9. Do you start your day with a cup of coffee for an energy boost?   Yes or No

10. Do you have a bowel movement late in the day or sometimes skip a day?   Yes or No

11. When you come home from work, are you exhausted?   Yes or No

12. Do you get a second wind around 10 p.m. and then stay up late watching TV or get on your computer?   Yes or No

13. Do you feel too tired and stiff to exercise in the morning?   Yes or No

14. Do you feel moody or melancholy in the winter or around the holidays?   Yes or No

15. Do you dread Monday mornings?   Yes or No

Now go back and look at the questions you answered "Yes" to. These are areas in your life where you may have a circadian clock imbalance.

In this chapter, my goal is to help create a lifestyle that can reset your circadian clock, because much more than your digestion depends on it.

Circadian Rhythms 101

Circadian rhythms are the light and dark cycles of the day that are as old as the very first cellular life forms on Earth.[268, 269] Both ancient Ayurvedic wisdom and modern science agree that living and eating in sync with nature's cycles is of utmost importance to our health, well-being, and even our longevity.[267] In fact, new research is suggesting that circadian "clocks" in the skin—which line the body, sense organs, and digestive and respiratory tracts—play a vital role in human health, immunity, cellular regeneration, and digestion.[267, 270]

There are numerous circadian clocks in the human body that sense and deliver regulatory messages regarding everything from when foods are harvested, to when we should eat and digest them. High concentrations of our circadian clocks are found throughout the digestive system, and research is proving the importance of following the circadian cycles of nature in order to optimize our digestive strength and health.[267]

For example, studies reveal when people disrupt their circadian rhythms with a stressful lifestyle that disregards the body's circadian clocks, such as frequent jet lag or late night shift work, they are more vulnerable to a variety of chronic digestive-related ailments.[271]

Do you indulge in late-night snack-fests? If you are in the habit of eating late at night, yet your 2-million-year-old clock is oriented to eating in the daytime, your body, its microbes, and even its genes can lose the ability to hear and sync up with nature's circadian rhythms. Over time, this dials down digestive strength and the ability to digest foods like wheat and dairy effectively, putting you at risk for more serious health issues.[272-274]

Eating bigger meals for breakfast and lunch along with a lighter supper—a concept based on circadian rhythms—as opposed to eating a heavy dinner or multiple mini meals throughout the day, delivers a host of health benefits including better digestion, more balanced blood sugar and blood pressure levels, and potential weight loss.[275-277]

When you are out of sync with the circadian rhythms, the gut bacteria responsible for regulating digestion of wheat and dairy, stabilizing your mood, cognitive function, immunity, blood sugar, detoxification and longevity, are also compromised.[271]

This was profoundly demonstrated when a group of healthy individuals flew from the U.S. to Israel and back, nonstop. When they returned, their gut bugs had gone from normal to microbes typically seen in diabetes and obesity.[271]

In the same study, when they disabled the circadian clock in a group of healthy nocturnal mice, the mice began eating all day instead of at night. Like the human group, their microbes shifted from healthy to what is more common in obesity and diabetes.

Additionally, when the researchers transplanted some of the jet-lagged human fecal matter into a new group of healthy mice, mice began to eat nonstop during the day instead of at night, and had the same microbe disturbance as the jet-lagged human group and mice without a circadian clock.[271]

Quick Tips to Start Improving Digestion

- **Tip 1:** Take time to eat a relaxing, balanced meal for lunch. If possible, make this the biggest meal of the day. Eat heavier and harder-to-digest foods like wheat and dairy during this time.

   Eating a heavy meal laden with bread and dairy in the evening, when the body's digestive clock has been turned off, may render these foods as undigested intestinal irritants and raise your blood sugar.[275-277]

- **Tip 2:** Make an effort to get to bed early and get up as close to or before the sunrise as possible. Regular sleep habits—including going to bed early and not working into the wee hours of the night—are linked to better digestion, optimal health and a longer life. Try your best to get 7–8 hours of sleep each night to stay in rhythm with the circadian clocks.[278-280]

Gluten and Dairy are Seasonal Foods

Every spring, which I like to call "nature's new year," a new stable of microbes are established in the lining of the digestive tract.[281-284] The rumen (the first chamber of the stomach) found in herbivores, such as cattle, is populated by microbes that are equipped to digest the bitter roots and fresh leaves of spring. This springtime microbial population changes so that in winter, different microbes predominate that aid in digesting the tougher wood fibers, nuts, seeds, tubers and grains; the true seasonal foods of the cold months. In turn, with the changing of the seasons, these winter microbes are once again replaced by a new population of microbes that digest the greens and emerging fruits of spring and summer. [282, 284, 285]

If we ate the way nature intended, a similar microbial adjustment would take place in our human digestive systems. Eating seasonally provides a subtle yet powerful shift in microbiology needed to effectively digest seasonal foods like wheat and dairy.

Let's see what happens in nature when a deer eats out of season. Let me share a quote from the book *The Forest Unseen* by David George Haskell to illustrate this point: [282]

"If a deer is fed corn or leafy greens in the middle of winter, [out of season] its rumen will be knocked off balance, acidity will rise uncontrollably, and gases will bloat the rumen. Indigestion of this kind can be lethal." [282]

In other words, when an herbivore eats foods that are not in season, it causes a drastic shift in its microbiology, leading to severe indigestion that can actually *kill* the herbivore. Cows, for example, when taken from pastures and fed grain instead of seasonal grasses, have to be medicated to settle their stomachs. [286]

If eating foods that are not in season can kill a deer and make a cow sick, [282] then perhaps this a is message for us to begin to respect the diet that has been right in front of us all these years—the diet that follows the harvests of nature!

Without a diet rich and diverse in seasonally-changing foods and microbes, our intestines are often populated by out-of-season microbes [287] which prevent us from gleaning the full health and digestive benefits of syncing up with nature's rhythms. Without the influx of seasonal microbes to boost our digestive strength and support a diverse community of essential and beneficial bacteria, we can become extremely vulnerable and often hypersensitive to our environment and foods. [288]

Foods like wheat, soy, nuts, seeds, and other grains are generally harvested in the fall, and offer a higher protein and fat nutrient content, which is required to help insulate for the cold winter months. The key here is in understanding that our ancestors ate foods such as gluten and dairy during the cold months, because that's the only time when these foods are available or ripe in nature—they were never intended to be eaten year-round with every meal.

Digestive Strength Increases in Winter

Modern research confirms what the ancient health science of Ayurveda has known for thousands of years—digestive strength gets stronger in the winter. For instance, one study found that amylase, a digestive enzyme in the body that breaks down sugar and wheat, increases in response to cold winter weather. Wheat has natural amylase inhibitors that protect the grain from digestion. Human digestion figured out a way to get around this by increasing the production of amylase during the cold winter months. A lack of amylase has been linked to wheat allergies and baker's asthma in one study, suggesting that a portion of the wheat allergies are due to sugar intolerance rather than gluten intolerance.[67] The parasympathetic vagal response—the body's rest-and-digest nervous system response that activates and facilitates digestion—also gets a boost in cold winter months.[70] Connected to the circadian rhythms, the body naturally boosts its own ability to digest the foods that are seasonally available.[70]

Increasing the digestive fire in the winter, according to Ayurveda, also has the effect of helping warm the body during the colder winter months. The opposite is also true. In the summer, the body is wired to help dissipate heat as a survival tool, and thus the digestive strength naturally decreases. Luckily, the summer harvest of mostly fruits and vegetables is cooked on the vine all summer by the hot sun, and thus, in a sense, are predigested and, therefore, not as much digestive fire is required. Of course, this works great if you live on a farm and are eating off the land, but if your summer diet is rich in burgers, fries, barbeque and milkshakes, your summer digestive strength may not be enough to efficiently break down these foods.

The Longevity Lifestyle

Dream a little dream with me. Imagine enjoying a meal with wheat and dairy with no unwanted side effects...

- Imagine finishing your day with the same energy you started with.
- Imagine going through your day without craving sweets, coffee, or chips.
- Imagine waking up early without an alarm, refreshed and ready to go.
- Imagine feeling like your life is not a struggle—like the wind is at your back and you are floating joyfully downstream on the river of life.

These are not pipe dreams; they are the reality of living with awareness and in connection with the cycles of nature—the benefits of syncing up with nature's circadian rhythms is well-supported by the new science of circadian medicine.[289]

Nature's Cycles According to Ancient Wisdom and Circadian Science

In nature, according to Ayurveda and similar principles in traditional Chinese medicine, there are two 12-hour cycles that are each divided into 3 smaller cycles. Each 4-hour cycle is linked to certain bodily functions governed by one of the following:

- **Vata** *(air element)*, which controls the nervous system
- **Pitta** *(fire element)*, which controls digestion and metabolism
- **Kapha** *(earth and water elements)*, which controls immunity and structural strength

According to Ayurveda, the daily lifestyle flow that syncs the body with nature's rhythms, and is also backed by circadian science,[289] is as follows:

First 12 Hours of the Day: 6 a.m.–6 p.m.

- **6 a.m.–10 a.m.** Kapha increases, corresponding to the earth and water elements and the seasons of late winter and early spring. This is the best time for exercise and physical labor before the sun is at its peak heat. This is a heavy time of day, illustrated by the stiffness and dullness you may experience when you sleep in. This heaviness, if you are up when the sun rises, supports greater physical strength. Eat a good-sized breakfast during this time, as it not only provides you with a reliable source of fuel for the day, but it will also help reduce obesity and disease.[290-293]

- **10 a.m.–2 p.m.** Pitta increases, corresponding to the fire element and the seasons of late spring into summer. This is the best time to relax and eat the biggest meal of the day because your digestive fire is at its strongest, hottest, and brightest in the middle of the day, just like the sun overhead at noon.[294] Eating earlier in the day, including a good breakfast and lunch, has been linked to numerous health benefits, including reduced cholesterol and stress.[291] Not only that, but the nutrient blueprint of the vegetables we eat is most potent at noon; a perfect nutritional gift from nature.[295, 296] Around noon is also the best time to digest foods like wheat and dairy.

- **2 p.m.–6 p.m.** Vata increases, corresponding to the air and ether elements and the seasons of fall and winter. This is the best time for mental and creative energy, as your nervous system is more active at this time of day. Craving sweets or caffeine at this time indicates exhaustion, blood sugar issues, poor digestion, or that you didn't eat a sufficient lunch. Early evening is the best time for a light supper, as heavy foods do not digest well.[297]

Second 12 Hours of the Day: 6 p.m.–6 a.m.

- **6 p.m.–10 p.m.** Kapha increases, corresponding to the earth and water elements and the seasons of late winter and early spring. This is the "heavy" time of day, cortisol levels drop, and it's the ideal time to begin settling down for sleep.[298]

- **10 p.m.–2 a.m.** Pitta increases, corresponding to the fire element and the seasons of late spring into summer. This is the best time to be sleeping. Both the lymph channels of the brain—and ultimately the liver—engage in detox at this time (like a janitor cleaning floors and windows). If you are constantly up and awake during this time, the body's natural detoxification process is disturbed.[5, 299]

- **2 a.m.–6 a.m.** Vata increases, corresponding to the air and ether elements and the seasons of fall and winter. The nervous system begins to stir before the sun rises. This is the best time to sleep deeply and naturally wake up before the sunrise.[300-302] In traditional cultures, sunrise was when you started the workday and predawn was reserved for bathing, yoga, meditation and prayer.

When to Sleep

Imagine you went to bed tonight at midnight and woke up tomorrow morning at 10 a.m. How would you feel? In my seminars, when I ask this question (barring teenagers from answering), most folks say they would feel stiff, groggy, and as if they slept too much.

Imagine the next night, you went to bed at 8 p.m. and woke up at 6 a.m. How would you feel in comparison? Most folks say without hesitation that they would feel more rested, alert, awake, flexible, and as if they got a great night's sleep.

Surprisingly, both nights' sleep were 10 hours each. How you feel from these 2 different nights' sleep is not only about how much sleep you got; it's all about *when* you got it. This is an example of the difference between living in sync with your circadian cycles or going against them.

What to Eat

With farmers' markets, farm shares, and community-supported agriculture (CSA) programs, eating seasonally and sourcing fresh-baked sprouted and fermented breads has never been easier. Traditionally, before the industrial age, folks were *forced* to only eat local and seasonally; we now have a choice. This can also be our downfall. The key is to include as many fresh, organic seasonal foods into your diet as possible.

Ayurvedic medicine, however, has made seasonal eating far from austere. Ayurveda classifies all the foods from around the world into grocery lists from each of the 3 harvests in nature. There are grocery lists based on nature's 3 primary harvests: Spring, summer and fall/winter. You can find the 3 seasonal grocery lists in my book, *The 3-Season Diet,*[294] in Appendix A of this book, and also on my website at LifeSpa.com.

⫸⫸⫸ ———————————————————————— ⫷⫷⫷

Instead of thinking about what you cannot eat in each season, think about what seasonal foods you can eat *more* of.

⫸⫸⫸ ———————————————————————— ⫷⫷⫷

Once the digestive system is stronger, the wheat you eat is a healthy variety, the bread is not processed, and the body's lymphatic channels are decongested, you will gain significant digestive wheat-eating strength.

A key to begin repairing your digestive power is to eat the foods that are harvested in each season and eat less of the foods not on the seasonal grocery list. Seasonal foods are nature's prescription for optimal health. Nutrient rations change, and the microbes in the soil and on the foods we eat change from one season to the next. As a result, the body's microbes—which make up 90 percent of the body's cells[66]—are adjusting seasonally to optimize its performance.

Using the lists is easy—circle the foods you are fond of in that season, and eat more of those seasonal foods. The foods marked with an asterisk are considered the superfoods of that season, and are extra beneficial in supporting your health.

Here is a basic guide to follow in planning your meals:

- 50 percent of the plate should be green vegetables
- 25 percent of the plate should be a protein (nuts, seeds, legumes, beans, dairy, meat and fish)
- 25 percent of the plate should be a starch (starchy root veggies like potatoes, beets, carrots, fruits, whole grains)
- As your digestion improves, the amount of food you will need will decrease and the types of foods you will choose will naturally change. Over time, try to limit the amount of animal protein you consume and replace it with plant-based proteins—all of which are naturally high in good fats. If you are a meat eater, aim to eat 10 percent of the total calories as animal meats.

- Add or cook with organic oils like ghee, coconut oil, or butter, and add organic extra virgin olive oil to the meal.
- Increase the amount of fat and protein intake during the colder winter months. This will happen naturally when you use the seasonal grocery lists.

When to Eat

As discussed earlier in this chapter, you can sync up with your circadian clock by eating 3 relaxing and balanced meals each day, with no snacking. Do your best to make lunch the biggest meal and eat an early, light supper.

The word supper is derived from the French word "souper," which means soup. Supper was historically a small supplemental meal, such as a soup.

We do much better when we eat the majority of our food in the daylight hours and minimal amounts at night. While eating at night has become the norm, it wasn't long ago that folks ate dinner at 4 and 5 o'clock. To demonstrate the risks of eating multiple meals throughout the day and night, one study compared eating just 2 meals a day, at breakfast and lunch, versus eating 6 small meals throughout the day and into the evening. The group that ate only breakfast and lunch had a significant reduction in body weight and fasting blood sugar levels, increased insulin sensitivity, and less fatty deposits in the liver. Both groups in the study ate the same amount of calories, but saw major differences in how the body responded to these 2 diets. Of course, the amount of food and the quality of food you eat does matter, but *when* you eat also plays a major circadian role in our health and well-being.[275]

I will delve deeper into the difference between eating 3 meals a day versus grazing throughout the day in Chapter 11, where I will teach you how to be a better fat burner.

How to Eat

There is an old saying that goes, "If you eat standing up, death looks over your shoulder." Around the world, for as long as we have recorded history, eating has been a sacred event, until now. Today, it seems that if you are not watching TV, checking Facebook, texting, or flipping through a magazine, the meal is somehow unsatisfying. Do your best to make eating a special time of your day, and plan ahead as to where and when you will be getting your 3 balanced meals that day. Eating on the run or while stressed activates the fight-or-flight sympathetic nervous system, which literally turns off digestive function. Being relaxed and calm while you eat increases the rest-and-digest parasympathetic nervous system that turns on digestion.[203]

Back in the late eighties, when I co-directed Deepak Chopra's Ayurvedic center, we had many seriously and terminally ill patients come to our clinic. They would stay for 1–2 weeks of detox and yoga, and would learn to meditate, spend time in nature, and eat gourmet Ayurvedic food.

At the end of everyone's stay, I would always ask the same question: "What was the most important thing you learned here this week?" I always expected them to tell me how they fell in love with the Ayurvedic massages or yoga, but the one thing I heard over and over again—and remember, these were mostly cancer patients—was that they were able to sit down, relax, stop, and actually enjoy the process of eating their food. They would tell me that in their everyday lives, eating had always felt like they were fueling their car—fill it up and go.

When you are trying to digest food, it makes a huge difference if you engage the parasympathetic nervous system.[203] Sitting down in a relaxed way allows the senses to smell, taste, and experience the food—all of which are linked to initiating the digestive process.

Chewing also seems to be an overrated concept for our fast-paced modern times. Meals are blended, fruits are juiced, and everything is gulped down on the run. While chewing is well-known for its benefits on digestion, few realize that chewing your food actually helps to relieve stress, boost mood, and enhance cognitive function and attention.[303, 304] The process of chewing seems to relax the nervous system by activating a parasympathetic response, which is what turns on the digestive process.[203] So before you inhale your next meal on the run, do your best to sit down and enjoy the process of chewing and eating your food.

Do We Eat Too Much?

Researchers have been searching for answers to the rise of obesity in America that is now reaching 1/3 of the population. Obesity is linked to what is called metabolic syndrome, which is a combination of abdominal obesity, high blood pressure, high blood sugar, high triglyceride levels, and low HDL cholesterol levels. Many experts have blamed gluten for the rise in obesity and the increase in metabolic syndrome.

In a large study published in the journal *Nutrition Research and Practice,* they compared American dietary trends from 1970–2008 as they relate to obesity. Researchers saw no associated trends with wheat and dairy. They did, however, find a link between bioengineered corn that is pervasive in our food chain, often showing up as high-fructose corn syrup, and linked to rising obesity levels.[305]

I am sure there is a new diet trend on the horizon condemning all corn in the way wheat has been condemned. Many foods will be blamed for our food intolerances, but it is more likely the *processed* nature of those foods and the fact that we have overeaten them along with a weak digestion that is the true culprit.

Not surprisingly, researchers also found a correlation between rising obesity levels and lack of physical activity. I will address our epidemic lack of physical activity and its relation to lymphatic congestion and gluten-related symptoms in upcoming chapters on lymph and exercise.[306]

Some studies suggest that this trend could be due to the increased portion sizes. According to the *American Journal of Public Health,* the amount of kilocalories (kcal) per day in the U.S. has increased by 500 kcal since the 1970s. That's almost a 25 percent increase in food consumption; very similar to the almost 33 percent obesity levels in America.[307]

Interestingly, Starbucks opened in 1971[308] and introduced Frappuccinos® in 1995.[309] America's 2015 favorite 16 ounce Grande Frappuccino® is the Caramel Cocoa Cluster, which weighs in with a whopping 470 calories and 75 grams of sugar.[310] I won't tell you how much is in a 24 ounce Venti® size. Okay, I will... it has 590 calories and 97 grams of sugar![310]

One of the most effective solutions for obesity, metabolic syndrome, and living a longer life is called "calorie restriction"—which is basically eating less.[306] Wheat, in this case, is guilty as charged. It has no doubt been over-consumed, over-produced, and over-processed.

Although portion control may be difficult at first, once you begin to eat balanced meals in harmony with your circadian rhythms your digestion will improve, your body will become more efficient at burning fat and you will find you feel satisfied with less food.

Mini Case Studies from the Office of Dr. John

I remember a patient, Sally[4], who came to see me for weight gain, digestive issues, and some bouts of depression. She came in for a follow-up visit in April of that year and was complaining that she had lost her appetite. Sally said her weight was down, her mood was much better, and that she was feeling great, except all she wanted was salad. In fact, she was craving it.

After thoroughly evaluating her, I came to the conclusion that it was springtime, and the seasonal harvest is comprised of spring greens and spinach salads—she was craving exactly what she *should* be craving. Eating less should not be something you have to will yourself to do. It should be something that comes quite naturally when your digestion is healthy.

I had a similar experience with Danielle[5], who came to see me for digestive issues. When Danielle came back in for a follow-up visit, she was clearly not happy. I first asked her about her abdominal pain, and she said that her digestion was feeling much better and that the pain was gone. She then told me that she lost her taste for coffee and she had just bought a very expensive espresso machine and now had no use for it. I reminded her that I didn't tell her to get off coffee and that the body will naturally adjust to craving and eating what it needs once the digestion is balanced. Although her abdominal pain was gone, she was still not happy about her new distaste for coffee!

---

4   All names of patients have been changed throughout this book to protect their privacy, and all patients have given permission to share the story of their health journey in this book.

5   All names of patients have been changed throughout this book to protect their privacy, and all patients have given permission to share the story of their health journey in this book.

Eating less may be the most powerful digestive health tool of all, but let's allow it to be a natural process. Back in 1935, the first paper on calorie restriction was published, which suggested that lifespans would be extended and diseases could be avoided by restricting calories without hunger or starvation.[311]

In the most comprehensive study on calorie restriction to date, which spanned 20 years, the results were nothing short of amazing. The study divided Rhesus monkeys into 2 groups. One group ate naturally without restraint and the other group ate a diet that was 30 percent lower in calories than the unrestricted group.[312]

After 20 years, 30 percent of the unrestricted diet group had died and only 13 percent of the calorie-restricted group had died from age-related illness. This translates into an almost three-fold reduction risk in age-related diseases.[312]

The monkeys that were calorie restricted had half the incidence of heart disease as the controls. Not one monkey in the calorie restricted group got diabetes, while 40 percent of the monkeys that ate as much as they wanted became diabetic or pre-diabetic.[312]

It works for humans too! When a group of adults reduced their calorie intake by only 20 percent for 2–6 years, blood pressure, blood sugar, cholesterol and weight were all significantly improved.[313]

Looking at all the research, it is hard to find any other intervention that has such compelling benefits on health and longevity than eating just 20–30 percent less food. An added bonus: When food and sugar levels are low, the cells live longer and the mitochondria of the cells make more energy in the form of ATP.[314, 315]

We clearly have the genetics to live long and healthy without an excess of food. The key is in the *kind* of fuel we are burning. Sugar, not wheat, is the underlying cause of much of our current health concerns.[101, 316, 317] As a result of the damaging health effects of overeating simple carbohydrates and sugar, we have lost the ability to burn fat. I will expand upon this in Chapter 11.

Strategies for Stronger Digestion and Eating Less

According to Harvard professor Daniel Lieberman, when we compare ancient humans to modern humans, ancient humans ate about 35 percent of their diet as carbs, including wheat, and we now eat around 45 percent. At first blush, not a big increase. However, for our ancestors, only 2 percent of those carbs were sugars, compared to our 30 percent! Ancient humans also ate about 100 grams of fiber per day, compared to our 15–20 grams.[257] Here are some dietary strategies to start eating less, naturally:

1. Eat More Good Fats

Sugars burn fast and quickly, leaving you wanting more. That makes it difficult to reduce calorie intake by 20–30 percent if your diet includes a lot of simple carbs and sugar. Ancient humans also ate a much higher percentage of good fats. Fat is actually the body's genetically preferred source of fuel—not sugar. One way to help cut back on the calories is to eat more good fats and reduce your intake of sugar and simple carbs (including processed breads, cooked and refined oils, dressings, chips, crackers, and sweets). Reducing sugar and refined carbs is a prerequisite before you start increasing fats.

One of my favorite ways to add healthy fats to my diet is to eat 1 teaspoon of very fresh, raw organic coconut oil with each meal, to help cut cravings. Once the cravings are gone after about a month, reduce this down to 1 teaspoon per day. I like to blend it into my hot tea every morning. This will deliver ketones (fat fuel) to the brain in minutes, and allow the brain to quickly get the message that we are full and less food is required.

I discuss beneficial fats and oils in more detail in Chapter 7.

2. Eat More Fiber

Increasing fiber in the form of beans and veggies will also help trigger a sense of fullness, so you can more easily leave the table with 20–30 percent fewer calories. When you evaluate the centenarian cultures around the world, there is 1 food group that they eat with breakfast, lunch, and dinner that they attribute their health and longevity to—beans.

Beans are loaded with nutrition and fiber. In fact, to even come close to eating 100 grams of fiber per day like our hunter-gatherer ancestors would be almost impossible to do without beans. Beans also support healthy blood sugar, heart health, balanced weight, and much more.[318-322] They are the ultimate high-fiber food.

While beans can be hard for some people to digest, there is one bean, according to Ayurveda, that is easily digestible and actually reduces gas—the split yellow mung bean. The hard-to-digest husk and anti-nutrient shell of the mung bean falls off during the splitting process. Whole mung beans have natural anti-inflammatory and anti-flatulence factors. More on these beans in Chapter 8. Once we reboot your digestion, you can move on to other types of beans.

3. Drink Water Between Meals

When we are dehydrated, the signals to our brain often get translated as hunger signals, making us think we need a snack rather than reaching for the H_2O. Getting plenty of plain, pure, filtered, room temperature water between meals can mitigate cravings.

In one study with 50 overweight girls, researchers instructed them to drink about 16 ounces of water, 3 times a day, half an hour before breakfast, lunch and dinner. This was over and above their normal daily water intake. After 8 weeks, they saw a significant decrease in body weight and body mass index. They concluded that water consumption increased thermogenesis and weight reduction in overweight subjects.[323]

More Tips to Boost Digestion and Reintroduce Wheat and Dairy

- **Tip 1:** Drink 16 ounces of water 30 minutes before each meal.
- **Tip 2:** Sit down and relax during the meal.
- **Tip 3:** Take time to chew your food—put the fork down between bites.
- **Tip 4:** Eat to only 3/4 full—don't overeat.
- **Tip 5:** Sip hot water with lemon with each meal, if you like.
- **Tip 6:** Don't talk business when you eat.
- **Tip 7:** Don't eat when you are angry or upset. It's better to skip that meal.
- **Tip 8:** Do your best to eat freshly prepared, seasonal foods rather than leftovers.

- **Tip 9:** Sit and rest for 10 minutes after the meal or lay on your left side while digesting.
- **Tip 10:** Finish with a short post-meal walk.
- **Tip 11:** Plan ahead for your next meal.
- **Tip 12:** Reduce all added sweeteners and take 1 teaspoon of raw organic coconut oil each day.
- **Tip 13:** Aim for 50 grams of fiber in your diet each day. Make half your plate green vegetables, 25 percent starch and 25 percent protein. Eat more beans. Start with easy-to-digest split yellow mung beans.
- **Tip 14:** Introduce small amounts of dairy and wheat during the mid-day meal and avoid these foods in the evening at the dinner meal.*
- **Tip 15:** Start with raw, organic cheese and/or ancient wheat or artisan sourdough bread. More on this in Chapter 7.*

Note: You may need to reboot digestion in Chapters 7-14 before starting wheat and dairy.

A Circadian Boost

If you are under regular stress, frequently crossing time zones, or living in contrast to the body's internal clocks and a lifestyle change is not possible at this time, consider some protective adaptogenic herbal support to help the body stay connected with the circadian rhythms to support optimal health, strong digestion, longevity, and well-being.[324]

Certain Ayurvedic herbs can boost digestive strength by helping to reconnect the body's internal clocks with the natural circadian rhythms. In one study, the herb *Bacopa monnieri* was found to support a healthy connection to the circadian rhythms while under significant oxidative stress.[325]

Bacopa,[325, 326] along with ashwagandha[327] and turmeric,[328-330] are all called brain-derived neurotrophic factors. These herbs support brain and mood function as well as the healthy regeneration of nerve cells when under stress.

Circadian Rhythms and Our Little Green Friends

It's not just humans who are affected by the circadian rhythms—it's every life form, including plants! As a part of the circadian cycles, every plant attracts a specific set of beneficial microbes from the soil, creating a symbiotic relationship between the plant and the microbes.[285, 331] Plants seem to benefit from certain microbes, and certain microbes seem to benefit from the nutrients of certain plants.

With each seasonal shift, the microbiology of the soil changes, the chemistry of the plants change, and the microbes that attach themselves to the roots, stems and leaves of each plant shift like the changing of the guard.[282, 285, 331, 332]

This matters to us because when we eat foods in season, we consume seasonal nutrients and seasonal microbes that deliver seasonal benefits for the body to stay healthy in each season. Nature's bounty is the perfect antidote to support our health in any season.

Looking Ahead

In Chapter 7, we will explore how to navigate the many choices to make regarding modern wheat and how we can still enjoy gluten products consciously, healthfully and safely.

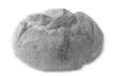

Chapter 7
NAVIGATING AROUND
MODERN TOXINS
IN OUR FOOD

A s I mentioned in Chapter 1, a major reason for the surge in gluten sensitivity is the *amount* of wheat we have been eating for the past 50–60 years. In 1961, American agronomist Norman Borlaug introduced the first high-yield wheat crop. Thanks to large amounts of fertilizers, his wheat was loaded with wheat berries, and soon his strain of high-yield wheat became the norm. The gluten content of his wheat, compared to the ancient wheat, is a topic of debate. However, it is clear that among higher-yield crops, wheat becomes less nutritious.[333, 334]

When wheat—a seasonal grain traditionally harvested only once a year—became hybridized, more processed, and started being harvested a couple times per year, the sugar content—or what is known as the glycemic index—of the wheat rose significantly.[335] And when we, as a culture, started eating wheat in excess, this became a real problem for our health.[336]

Gluten, Gluten Everywhere

Gluten became the staple that appeared in one form or another in almost every American meal year-round. It's in breakfast cereals, pancakes, sandwich breads, cakes, biscuits, pasta, pizza, rye crackers, multigrain chips, sausages, soya sauce, salad dressings, bouillon cubes, beer, modified food starch (present in many baby foods), canned soups, sauces, and textured vegetable proteins found in veggie burgers and the like.

Clearly, we have overshot the gluten runway and the amount of gluten we eat must be dialed down. Getting back to the traditional ways that humans ate and prepared wheat for thousands of years will allow our digestive tracts to heal from overeating this food.

Perhaps the most profound deviation from our healthier wheat-eating traditions is the shortened fermentation time of bread. As bread became more and more in demand, the process time, going from flour to loaf, shortened from days to just 2 hours. There are even commercial "no-time" bread doughs fermented for as little as zero–15 minutes.[337]

Fermentation: The Magic of Sourdough

When water and wheat flour are allowed to sit, they start to lacto-ferment. In the fermentation process, the lactobacilli—probiotic microbes naturally found on wheat—begin to ferment and eat the sugars and the gluten in the wheat. This naturally lowers the glycemic index of the wheat as well as lowers the gluten content significantly.[77, 338]

In one study published in 2007, research showed that sourdough bread made with wheat can be gluten-free. When sourdough bread is produced with a particular strain of lactobacilli, it was shown to have gluten levels of 12 parts per million (ppm). Anything less than 20 ppm is considered gluten-free. Bread made with the same wheat, but without lacto-fermentation, had gluten levels of 75,000 ppm.[77]

Slow fermented sourdough bread can render the bread gluten-free.

In a number of studies, sourdough bread produced a lower surge in blood sugar than any other bread. For instance, in one study, folks with impaired glucose tolerance were fed either sourdough or ordinary bread. The sourdough bread produced a significantly lower glucose and insulin response. In the long, slow fermentation required to make sourdough bread, important nutrients such as iron, zinc, magnesium, antioxidants, folic acid and other B vitamins becomes easier for our bodies to absorb.[338]

In the process of preparing sourdough bread, gluten can be broken down and rendered virtually harmless for those with intolerance. In one small Italian study, celiac patients fed sourdough bread for 60 days had no clinical complaints, and their biopsies showed no changes in the intestinal lining.[339]

Bread from the grocery store or even the health food store can be a far cry from traditional bread made with a long fermentation process. Ideally, the ingredients of your bread should look like this: Organic wheat, starter, salt and water.

In contrast, here is an example of the ingredient list of a top-selling organic sourdough bread. See if you can spot the ingredients added to expedite the fermentation process.

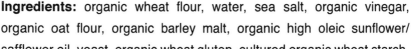

Ingredients: organic wheat flour, water, sea salt, organic vinegar, organic oat flour, organic barley malt, organic high oleic sunflower/safflower oil, yeast, organic wheat gluten, cultured organic wheat starch, organic whole wheat flour, ascorbic acid, natural enzymes.

The malt, oils, vinegar, starch, ascorbic acid and additional gluten are added to speed up the fermentation process, or needed to improve flavor. Remember, it's the naturally slow process of traditional fermentation that breaks down the gluten and grain anti-nutrients like phytic acid. A long fermentation time is also what gives traditional bread-baking its amazing aroma and flavor. In sharp contrast, if you ever get near an industrial bread plant, the aroma is almost nauseating.

This top-selling-brand bread—with the long ingredient list, above—is actually one of the better commercial breads on the market. But here are some telltale problems: It will still stay soft and fresh on the counter for weeks before growing mold, and perhaps never get hard like bread in the old days would do.

Try googling "organic, artisan, fermented breads" for your town and locate a baker who has traded in all the processing aids for traditional long fermentation, yielding low-glycemic bread. As another option, Manna Organics is a bakery that sells organic sourdough bread that you can order online, which only contains flour, water and salt.

While there are many artisan bakeries popping up all over the country making breads using ancient wheats and employing longer fermentation times, learning how to bake your own low-glycemic, low-gluten bread is a fun family project. I recommend using a Dutch oven to bake your bread. Le Creuset and Lodge are great brands, as they don't contain aluminum.

Note: In Appendix B, I have included 2 sourdough bread recipes. One is an old world sourdough bread recipe from a traditional bakery in Lourdes, France that was given to me by my mother from her days living in Europe and the other is a recipe from the master baker, Cathy Ligenza at the Kripalu Center for Yoga and Health in Lenox, Massachusetts where I regularly teach. Her bread is rare and the best I have ever tasted. We are all so lucky to have both these traditional sourdough recipes.

Sprouted, Soaked, Fermented Grains

Grains are dormant seeds that are awaiting the ideal environment to germinate and sprout into wheat, rice, barley, or oat cereal grass. All grains, as well as beans, have anti-nutrients such as phytates and enzyme inhibitors that allow the seed to lie dormant all winter and then germinate in the wet, moist, warmer spring.

These phytates are difficult to digest for some people. Studies have shown that soaking, sprouting or allowing the grain to germinate increases an enzyme called phytase that breaks down the phytates in wheat, other grains and legumes.[48] This renders the grain or bean much easier to digest for those who have weaker digestion. Fermenting the grains as is done when making sourdough bread, will do the same. Many artisan bakers, as in our *Eat Wheat* sourdough bread recipes will both soak and ferment the flour before baking.

When the digestive system is weak then soaking, fermenting or sprouting grains not only neutralizes the phytic acids as well as certain enzyme inhibitors like wheat germ agglutinin (WGA) present in all seeds, it encourages the production of numerous beneficial enzymes. The action of these enzymes also increases the amounts of many vitamins, especially B vitamins.

For the seed to germinate and sprout, it requires a burst of growth energy that uses up a significant amount of the starch in the grain. This can lower the sugar content in the sprouted grain and thus lower the glycemic index of grains that are soaked, germinated and sprouted.[50]

Some studies suggest that the vitamin, mineral, protein, fat and fiber content increases as a result of sprouting, but much of this increase is thought to be due to nutrient percentage changes as a result of the decreased starch content.[340]

Soaked and sprouted grains, legumes and breads are readily available in the marketplace or at your local artisanal bakery. Many health food store bakeries are employing these traditional techniques. Food for Life bread and Alvarado are 2 national brands that also make bread with sprouted grains. The telltale sign of a good quality bread is found in the ingredients. No cooked oils, no sweeteners, no additives. Just wheat (sprouted) water, salt and perhaps sourdough starter.

Phytic Acid Benefits

Phytic acids have been criticized based on studies suggesting they block the absorption of certain minerals such as iron, zinc, calcium and magnesium. There has been no consensus in the literature regarding mineral deficiencies from a high grain or phytic acid diet. While a certain amount of calcium absorption may be slowed, there are no findings linking this to bone density issues, and vegetarians who have the highest grain-based phytic acid diet do not seem to be mineral deficient as suggested.[341]

In fact, it seems the phytic acids in grains—which have been the mainstay of the diet for 3–4 million years—have many benefits, and their hard-to-digest nature may be part of a bigger, more important plan. For example, phytic acid slows down the absorption of sugars after a meal and thus is found to reduce cholesterol and triglycerides. It also reduces risk of hypercalcemia and kidney stones and has anti-colon cancer properties.[341]

Grains may not be the body's primary delivery system for minerals. That may be more of a function of vegetables and leafy greens. Wheat and other grains like barley, rye, spelt and oats are loaded with fiber. While oats and barley (a glutenous grain) are rich in soluble fibers, wheat is rich in insoluble fiber, and overall, one of the highest sources of fiber among all grains. Both the phytic acid and fiber content in wheat will both delay the absorption of certain nutrients and antioxidants in the small intestine, so they can be transported undigested to the colon where they feed the lion's share of the microbiology in the large intestine— who are truly responsible for our health, immunity, mood and digestion.[341]

In fact, in the large intestine, the fiber in wheat literally doubles the production of the short chain fatty acid, butyric acid, that is made from gut microbe fermentation. This is the same superfood fatty acid we talked about that is found in butter and ghee that supports intestinal health and detox. Increased butyric acid production from wheat fiber has been found to reduce tumor formation in the colon and protect the gut wall from cancer and intestinal damage.[341]

The antioxidants in the phytic acid have been shown to increase apoptosis, which is the accelerated death of colon cancer cells supporting the theory that there are great benefits from the phytic acids.[341] The most recent research suggests that these anti-nutrients, like phytic acids and indigestible insoluble fibers in wheat, are indigestible in the upper digestion to empower the lower digestion and beneficial microbes. Our sensitivity to phytic acid could simply mean that we just have some digestive strengthening to do.

WGA: Wheat Germ Agglutinin

WGA is a type of lectin or anti-nutrient found on wheat that protects it from insects and decay while the seed lies on the ground waiting for the spring thaw, to then germinate. Every grain and seed on the planet including rice, all beans, dairy and nightshades like tomatoes and potatoes have lectins and other anti-nutrients that protect them. It does not seem reasonable that we should avoid all grains and beans, as rice and beans have been a staple for humanity for thousands of years. When evaluating the diet of the centenarian cultures, who regularly live to over 100 years, they consume all of the above lectin-rich foods. Perhaps, we still have more to learn about the subtleties of the foods we eat.

While there are numerous studies labelling WGA and other lectins as toxic, inflammatory, neurotoxins, cancer-causing and a reason to avoid all grains,[59] some studies are beginning to change our understanding.

For example, one study demonstrated that the WGA has beneficial effects on the gastrointestinal tract and have anti-tumor properties. In fact, researchers are looking at WGA as a possible active ingredient for new anti-cancer drugs.[342]

As I mentioned, the complete understanding of how we digest wheat is a scientific work-in-progress. While evidence mounts against grains and WGA, there are compelling scientific arguments for grains. More compelling in my opinion is the breakdown of our digestive systems that will render us increasingly intolerant to many more foods in the future, if we do not address the underlying issues.

On the flip side, with the consumption of wheat being linked to the prevention of colon cancers, obesity, cardiovascular issues, diverticulitis disease, constipation and irritable bowel syndrome (IBS)[341] along with the fact that we have been digesting it for millions of years, it seems we are only beginning to understand wheat in its entirety.

Easier to Digest Gluten Grains

Spelt, which is a hardy, high-fiber variety of wheat, was found to have 40 percent less phytic acid content and more phytase activity when compared to a variety of common wheats. Spelt also had a significantly higher mineral content than most wheats, suggesting that spelt may be much easier to digest and a more nutritious variety of wheat to start with when we reintroduce wheat back into the diet.[343]

Rye bread has a lower glycemic load than regular wheat bread, suggesting that rye may also be a better choice for blood sugar control.[344, 345] Both rye and barley, which also contain gluten, have been shown to increase the production of butyric acid in the gut and thus support gut health and stable blood sugar. Crackers, such as the Wasa and Kavli brands, are made of rye, salt and water.

Barley is a glutenous grain that is rich in a slimy soluble fiber much like oatmeal, and in the same way oatmeal supports good heart health, so does barley. The fiber in barley called beta-glucan was shown to curb appetite and lower total cholesterol, LDL cholesterol and tryglycerides.[346] Beta-glucan is a slimy soluble fiber that blocks the absorption of sugars into the bloodstream. The barley fiber also attaches to and escorts toxic bile from the intestines to the toilet, which supports healthy gallbladder and liver function. The beta-glucan fiber in barley has also been found to prevent obesity, high blood sugar and metabolic syndrome—which is a combination of blood pressure, blood sugar and obesity concerns.[346]

The Benefits of Ancient Wheats

Using the right kind of flour makes a difference in the digestibility of the wheat. Studies have shown that ancient wheat is much simpler, genetically, than modern, hybridized wheat. For example, the oldest known type of wheat is called einkorn, and has just 14 chromosomes or 7 sets of diploids (pairings of 2 chromosomes). Durum wheat, used for most pastas, as well as emmer (also sometimes known as farro) and KAMUT® khorasan wheat—which are also ancient wheats—have 28 chromosomes and are known as tetraploid, meaning they contain pairings of 3 chromosomes. The wheat most commonly used in breads made from spelt has 42 chromosomes, which are known as hexaploid wheats, containing pairings of 6 chromosomes.[347]

Studies have shown that the wheats with more chromosomes have higher levels of gliadin, which is considered one of the more difficult components of the gluten to digest.[348]

In another study, researchers suggest that selecting your wheat based on these chromosomal factors can reduce the celiac immunogenic potential. In other words, if you have weak digestion, choose a wheat product with lower levels of chromosomes, which tend to be the more ancient wheats, where there will be lower levels of gliadin, and be easier to digest for folks who are sensitive to gluten.[349]

Many of the ancient tetraploid wheats (such as durum, emmer, and KAMUT® khorasan wheat) have been shown to have higher antioxidant potentials[350] and higher plant sterol profiles than the modern hexaploid wheats—both of these qualities are supportive of our health.[351] Plant sterols help support healthy cholesterol levels and heart health, possess anti-inflammatory qualities, and have even been linked to reducing the risk of cancer.[352]

With a strong digestive system and a healthy lining of intestinal skin, all of the non-processed wheats should be digestible unless, of course, there is a diagnosis of genuine celiac disease. Some are clearly better and easier to digest than others as a result of less hybridization. If you plan on eating a lot of wheat, the kind of wheat you choose matters, so shop carefully or bake your own. If you bake your own, Resurgent Grains is a great online resource for organic whole grain flour.

While ancient wheats are easier to digest, even modern wheat can be digested well by a strong digestive system. Sourdough bread made from modern wheat presents little to no problems, and true sprouted grain breads like Ezekiel 4:9 Sprouted 100 percent Whole Grain Bread by Food for Life, or Manna Breads® by Manna Organics, are much easier to digest as well.

A Word about Soy: Once a Toxin, Now a Food?

If you're confused about wheat and dairy, soy may be the most confusing hard-to-digest food of all. Ancient writings from China suggest that the soybean was traditionally considered unfit for human consumption. In China, the discovery that soy could be cultured or fermented brought a shift in soy's reputation. While unfermented soy was still avoided as a food, the fermentation process appeared to free soy from toxic anti-nutrients and, moreover, actually released some amazing health benefits.[353] During the Ming Dynasty, the fermented soy food, "natto," found its way into *Chinese Herbal Medicine: Materia Medica*,[354] as a nutritional remedy for many health conditions.

Today, many experts believe that fermentation, as seen in tempeh, natto, miso, and traditionally brewed soy sauce, is the only way to neutralize the dangerous anti-nutrients in soy.[355] Unfortunately, tofu, which is the most commonly consumed form of soy in the U.S., is not fermented. As a result, it is quite difficult to digest and commonly a cause of digestive concerns and food allergies.

Soybeans—as well as all beans, wheat, and most grains—are endowed with certain protective anti-nutrients that can be hard to digest.[356-358] Many plants are protected by toxic anti-nutrients to ward off insects and animals that might otherwise eat them. Beans, in particular, are famous for these anti-nutrients which, as many of us may know from experience, can make them a challenge to digest.

Unlike most beans, the anti-nutrients in soy[356-358] don't wash or cook off, and according to the research by soy opponents, they present significant health risks. What is clear, however, is much like with wheat, when soy is fermented, these anti-nutrients are broken down by bacteria, and soy becomes much easier to digest, as we saw with sourdough bread. That said, the anti-nutrients in wheat, like phytic acid, are much easier to digest than those in soybeans. A good, healthy digestive system can break down the anti-nutrients in wheat, even without fermentation. Always be sure to buy organic, non-GMO soy products.

Intestinal Damage From GMOs

An explosion in gluten sensitivity is affecting more than 18 million Americans today.[359] This may be explained, in part, by the introduction of genetically modified organisms (GMOs) into our food supply. GMOs are living organisms whose genetic material has been artificially manipulated in a laboratory through genetic engineering, or GE. This process creates combinations of plant, animal, bacterial and viral genes that do not occur in nature or through traditional crossbreeding methods. While wheat is not (yet) a genetically modified crop, new studies are finding an interesting link between the consumption of GMOs and today's rising rate of gluten intolerance.

GMOs were introduced into the American food supply in the mid-1990s. Today, there are 9 genetically modified food crops on the market in the U.S.:

1. Soy
2. Corn
3. Cotton (oil)
4. Canola oil
5. Sugar from sugar beets

6. Zucchini
7. Yellow squash
8. Papaya
9. Alfalfa

In addition, here's a list of common ingredients derived from GMO crops and found in processed foods (See www.nongmoproject.org):

- Amino Acids
- Aspartame
- Ascorbic Acid
- Sodium Ascorbate
- Vitamin C
- Citric Acid
- Sodium Citrate
- Ethanol
- Flavorings ("natural" and "artificial")
- High-Fructose Corn Syrup
- Hydrolyzed Vegetable Protein
- Lactic Acid
- Maltodextrins
- Molasses
- Monosodium Glutamate
- Sucrose
- Textured Vegetable Protein (TVP)
- Xanthan Gum
- Vitamins
- Yeast Products

Certain GMO crops are considered "Roundup Ready" meaning they have been genetically engineered to include the weed killer called Roundup, whose active ingredient is a known toxin—glyphosate. Roundup Ready crops include soy, corn, canola, alfalfa, cotton, and sorghum. Wheat is currently under development. In addition, Roundup is sometimes liberally sprayed on non-organic wheat and genetically modified crops to kill weeds and speed up the harvesting process.

Unfortunately, the companies that manufacture GMOs (such as Monsanto) have a very strong lobby presence in government, and legislation to require labeling of GMOs has been constantly defeated. GMOs are not required to be identified or labeled in any way. However, if you focus on eating only organic, or look for the "Non GMO Project" label, you can avoid the GMO versions of these foods.

Additionally, GMO sweet corn is genetically engineered to be both Roundup Ready and to produce its own insecticide called Bt toxin. As a result, this insecticide finds its way into all the non-organic, GMO corn products on the market, which are very difficult to avoid. For instance, every time you eat at a restaurant and the food is not organic, chances are you are ingesting some GMO corn residues, whether it be in their vegetable oil, corn syrup, corn starch, mayonnaise, ketchup, chips, tortillas, or corn itself.

Roundup on Your Wheat

What the vast majority of the public does not know is that in the past 15 years, it is a practice for wheat farmers in certain areas (primarily North and South Dakota and parts of Canada) to spray their wheat fields with Roundup or glyphosate several days before harvest. Monsanto, the manufacturer of Roundup, introduced this practice in the 1980s. For the farmer, spraying the wheat before harvest acts as a desiccant and helps dry—and ultimately kill—the wheat plant, which forces it to release more seeds. Even areas of the field that are still green will ripen quickly so the farmer can harvest a more uniform crop with a higher yield.[360]

Some experts are linking not only the epidemic of non-celiac gluten sensitivity to ingesting glyphosate, but also the dramatic increase in celiac disease. In a study published in the *Journal of Interdisciplinary Toxicology*, researchers found a strong correlation between celiac disease and the use of glyphosates. The chart below, illustrating the study's findings, shows a parallel trend of the increase use of glyphosate and the incidence of celiac disease.[62]

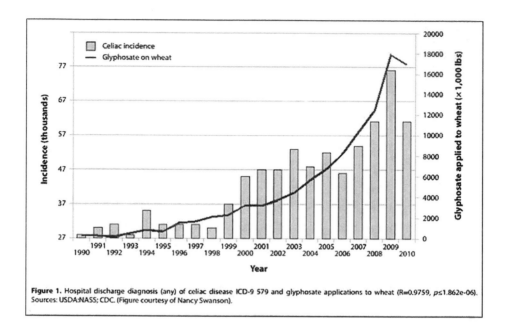

Figure 1. Hospital discharge diagnosis (any) of celiac disease ICD-9 579 and glyphosate applications to wheat (R=0.9759, p≤1.862e-06). Sources: USDA:NASS; CDC. (Figure courtesy of Nancy Swanson).

Casualties of GMOs—Killing Your Gut Bacteria

When glyphosate is ingested by eating GMO foods or non-organic foods that have been sprayed with Roundup, studies have measured the reduction of the good bacteria and the overgrowth of harmful strains of bacteria in the gut.[361] These strains have been shown to irritate the intestinal wall and be a possible contributor to the intolerance of gluten. Exposure to glyphosate is insidious, as it causes a slow, steady, gradual alteration of the gut microbiome and inflammation of the intestinal tract. Gut bacteria have been shown to aid in digestion, protect the intestines from permeability and autoimmune conditions, and boost immunity and synthesizing vitamins.[362]

The gut bacteria are also responsible for manufacturing certain amino acids that are essential to optimal health and digestion. Glyphosate has been shown to disturb the function of the gut microbes.[62] It has also been shown to inhibit the cytochrome P450 enzymes, which help break down other foreign chemicals, environmental toxins, and xenobiotics that are extremely toxic and inflammatory to the intestinal wall.

Research shows GMO foods decrease levels of the pancreatic enzyme precursor called zymogen, required for digesting hard-to-digest proteins. This study was done on mice who were fed farmed fish that were raised on GMO feed.[363] Without digestive enzymes, hard-to-digest proteins like gluten become much harder to digest.

The result of this long-term exposure is chronic intestinal and systemic inflammation of the body. The experts that have condemned gluten have blamed gluten on this epidemic of inflammation, but the science is clear that gluten is not the actual culprit.[62] The same conditions that science is now linking to GMO and glyphosate damage have been misappropriated to gluten.

To avoid glyphosate exposure: Buy organic wheat. I recommend ancient einkorn, emmer, KAMUT® khorasan wheat, or spelt, whenever possible.

But this alone is not enough—if you have food intolerances, you must also repair the damage to your intestines incurred from years of Roundup and GMO intestinal and digestive damage. See Chapter 8 for details and tips on how to accomplish this task.

The GMO Bt Toxin

The genetically engineered Bt toxin found in corn is designed to be toxic to many insect species found on crops, puncturing holes through the intestines of the insect. A new study has shown that Bt toxin can puncture holes through the human digestive tract as well![364] What's even worse is that Bt toxin is carried by pregnant moms and transmitted to the fetus, possibly predisposing infants to food intolerances.[365]

One of the suggested effects of gluten sensitivity is "leaky gut," or intestinal permeability into the lymphatic system, which we now know may be related to intestinal irritants such as Bt toxin.[62, 364]

Bt toxin has been shown to activate an immune response against foods that were previously digestible.[366] It is very possible that exposure to this insecticide in corn products may have activated an immune hypersensitivity response to hard-to-digest proteins such as gluten.

Gluten Sensitivity in Children and Infants

Food allergies in kids are very common and are often complex and difficult to treat. Simply taking kids off wheat and dairy only helps a small percentage of kids leaving the doctor's office. While I am by no means suggesting that I have all the answers to this problem, there are a few glaring concerns I'd like to mention.

Mineral and vitamin deficiencies are common in infants and children. Most common are vitamin D3 and iron. Both deficiencies can have a negative impact on the digestive function of a child.[367]

Infant formulas are often loaded with preservatives, sweeteners, and hard-to-digest ingredients like soy, corn maltodextrin (sugar), and a variety of highly processed oils that even most adults could not digest well. Children's digestive systems are very delicate, which is why traditional cultures often introduced foods to a child one at a time—very slowly—so as to nurse the digestion along until it develops its own healthy digestive and immune-boosting microbiome.

Mental, emotional and physical stress is also a factor that can disturb the microbiome of the baby. Even in utero, maternal stress has been shown to alter the development of the infant's microbiome. In fact, in one study, the stress of the mom during pregnancy was directly linked to an alteration of beneficial intestinal microbes and the early onset of food allergies and poor intestinal health in the child.[368] In Ayurveda, much attention is given to making sure the mother is as stress-free during her pregnancy as possible.

As we begin to understand the delicate nature of the microbiome, which I discuss fully in Chapter 8, we realize that emotional stress has a powerful impact on our digestive strength for both children and adults. For more on children's health, see my book, *Perfect Health For Kids.*[369]

Common Food Additives to Avoid

Additives found in many health foods have also been implicated in killing beneficial gut microbes and they can irritate and damage the intestinal wall directly. The first line of defense against experiencing sensitivity reactions to wheat or dairy is to maintain the health and function of the intestinal wall.

Commonly used emulsifiers have been found guilty of wreaking havoc on the intestinal skin, and thus our digestive function.[370-372]

Emulsifiers (such as polysorbate-80 and carboxymethyl cellulose) are everywhere—they are used in processed foods, drugs, vitamins, vaccines, soaps, and cosmetics. Their function is to keep oils and water from separating. They are found in everyday products ranging from mouthwash to ice cream, salad dressing to barbecue sauce.[373]

Researchers believe that constant low-grade irritation to the intestinal wall from these emulsifiers will ultimately disturb the microbiome, resulting in impaired digestion and blood sugar regulation, as well as an increased susceptibility to weight gain—*all classic symptoms of food intolerances.*[372]

With this new research trending, it is becoming clearer and clearer that if you don't recognize the name of an ingredient on a label, it may be something that the FDA recognizes as safe, but it still might be damaging your intestines as well as your microbiome, and play a large role in your food sensitivities and intolerances.

Carrageenan—a Safe Seaweed?

On first inspection, the food additive called carrageenan seems quite harmless. Derived from the edible red seaweed Chondrus crispus—commonly called Irish moss or carrageen moss—it has been used for some 600 years as a thickening agent for foods.[374]

Today, it is a popular vegetarian alternative to gelatin and is found in many common foods like almond, rice, soy and coconut milks, ice creams, cottage cheese, yogurts, creamers, salad dressings, desserts, sauces, diet sodas, processed meats, vegetarian meats, beers, toothpastes, and more.

The original research, performed back in 1982, cleared food-grade carrageenan as safe to use as a food additive.[375] But new evidence, which points out the flaws in those early studies, suggests that food-grade carrageenan may be a bowel irritant and potential carcinogen.[370, 371]

Based on a meta-analysis of many studies on the safety of food-grade carrageenan by Joanne Tobacman, M.D., there are documented toxic effects (bowel ulcerations) of the un-degraded (food-grade) carrageenan in humans. It was also shown to have a carcinogenic effect in animals.[371]

In Tobacman's thorough review, the studies suggest that the so-called safe un-degraded carrageenan is actually broken down into the degraded or toxic form of carrageenan by the digestive stomach acid.[370, 371]

If these studies are accurate, the food-grade carrageenan that is so common in the American diet may be responsible, in part, for many of the bowel inflammatory cases, gluten and dairy intolerances, and blood sugar concerns. In addition, carrageenan may also be acting as a silent carcinogen.[370, 371, 376]

Again, although this conclusion is not shared by the FDA and many food safety organizations in both the USA and the European Union, many companies are taking note and removing carrageenan from their ingredients as a result of public pressure.[377]

Avoid Cooked or Rancid Oils in Processed Foods

If you are buying bread, chips, crackers or cookies, you will likely see some type of oil in the ingredients. If that product has been cooked or baked, that oil has been rendered very difficult to digest. Even if the oil is organic and cold-pressed, once it has been heated, the more natural it is, the more quickly it goes rancid.

Rancid oils have a congestive effect on the function of the liver and gallbladder. As we have already discussed, if there is compromised bile flow, the stomach will be less likely to produce the required amount of acid needed to break down the proteins in wheat and dairy.

When you buy "cold-pressed" cooking oil, do you assume that the seeds were pressed safely at a cool temperature to protect the oil from rancidity, trans fats, and other toxic processing chemicals? Unfortunately, this couldn't be further from the truth.

The modern cold-pressing process heats the oil multiple times, rendering most oils either rancid or so sterile that there are no natural ingredients left to actually go rancid. Natural unrefined oils are so delicate that even minimal exposure to daylight will trigger a chain reaction of free radical damage, creating trans fats and other byproducts that experts believe to be even more harmful than trans fats![378] Traditionally, seeds were hand-pressed to make oils under very low temperatures and delivered to homes like milk—in dark amber bottles, due to the volatility of these oils.

"How can they sell cooking oils in clear plastic bottles that are exposed to the light?" you may ask. Well, they shouldn't; but they do because it's less expensive to produce and transport. Keep in mind these oils are used in industrial bread production to help keep it soft and squishy for weeks.

Refined, Bleached, and Deodorized Oils in Bread

Udo Erasmus, author of the book, *Fats That Heal, Fats That Kill*, states that, "After oils are pressed or solvent extracted from seeds and nuts, they are degummed, refined, bleached, and deodorized. The result is known as an RBD (refined, bleached, deodorized) and these oils, as a result, become colorless, odorless, and tasteless." [378]

In addition, valuable beneficial ingredients are removed during processing, including antioxidants, lecithin, chlorophyll and other beneficial molecules.

The oil is now dead! It is refined, odorless, tasteless, colorless, and void of most nutritional value. This is similar to the way the natural fats in milk are harmed by the high heat during the ultra-pasteurization process, or during homogenization when the fats are slammed through a tiny filter, making them homogenized, meaning "all the same size."

The Good Oils

According to Erasmus, most oils—except extra virgin olive oil—have been processed by these destructive methods. Extra virgin olive oil, while not overly damaged by processing, can be damaged by high heat in the cooking process. [378] Ideally, olive oil should not be used for cooking, but can be added to foods after they are removed from the heat.

Look for expeller-pressed (screw press) oils by manufacturers that make an effort to keep the pressing temperature low. A manufacturer concerned about overheating oils will mention expeller pressure temperature on the label. Look for pressing temperatures below 122°F, which is the European standard for cold (expeller) pressing. These oils are safe and desirable—but are not to be used for cooking! Also, look for harvest dates and press dates on the oils you buy. Unlike fine wine that gets better with age, oils do not. The antioxidant polyphenols in vegetable oils have a definite shelf life.

The best organic oils to safely use for cooking (the most heat tolerant) and their corresponding smoke point temperatures are: [379]

- Avocado oil—520°F
- Mustard oil—489°F
- Ghee—485°F
- Hazelnut oil—430°F
- Grapeseed oil—420°F
- Macadamia oil—413°F
- Coconut oil—350°F
- Butter—350°F

If It Doesn't Go Bad, Don't Eat It

Some of us remember buying bread from a bakery in the old days. If it wasn't eaten in a day or two, it would get hard or grow some mold. Today, as I discussed earlier, we have organic whole wheat bread that by all measures is sold as healthy bread, yet it will sit on the counter for weeks, stay soft, and not go bad. Remember, it is beneficial bacteria that makes bread spoil. So, if the bugs won't eat the bread on your counter, should you?

Think about the jars of condiments in your refrigerator that have been there for weeks, months, and maybe even years. Don't you wonder why it can stay in the fridge for so long and not spoil? Most of these jars of condiments have preservatives, or refined and processed oils that are resistant to growing any type of bacteria, good or bad.

We should be eating foods that will feed your microbes.[66] In general, your microbes love good fats and fiber. Microbes are not big fans of processed sugar, carbs, and processed oils in breads or milk.[66] In our culture, we have done a bang-up job of killing off many strains of microbes that are now recognized as being required for optimal health and digestion of gluten and dairy.

Consider throwing out all those items in your fridge that are older than a month or two. That is a good start.

Natural Preservation Methods

Of course, there are natural preservation methods such as lacto-fermentation, culturing dairy, and sugar and salt methods that actually employ the good bugs to keep undesirable bacteria away from these foods. As a result, many of these foods—like miso, kimchi, sauerkraut, and some kinds of cheeses—are quite healthy. Adding small amounts of lacto-fermented foods to your daily diet is a great way to feed the beneficial bugs in your gut.

Dried grains and beans—as well as dense root and ground vegetables like cabbage and beets—can naturally keep for longer than a month. Foods such as these take an entire season to grow and are naturally very hardy and resistant to spoilage.[380] Nature has its own way of preserving foods for the winter that we have been unable to artificially match. When cleaning out your fridge and cabinets, these foods can be the exception.

Looking Ahead

Now that we have discussed some of the ways to best navigate around the many toxins in our food supply and their deleterious effects on our health, it is time to run a fine tooth comb through every aspect of your digestive system and fix it.

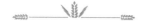

How to Fix Your Digestion

Next, to successfully reintroduce wheat and dairy back into the diet we must accomplish the following:

1. Repair the intestinal skin, establish regular elimination and repopulate the gut with permanent wheat- and dairy-digesting microbes. (Chapter 8)

2. Repair and decongest the lymphatic system that is responsible for most food intolerance symptoms in the brain and the body. (Chapter 9)

3. Troubleshoot and reboot every aspect of the upper digestion including stomach HCl production, the flow of bile and the production of pancreatic and duodenal enzymes. (Chapter 10)

4. Bring the blood sugar back into balance, which is the epidemic of our time. Unstable blood sugar can make you more vulnerable to grain-related sugar spikes and lows. (Chapter 11)

5. Reset digestive strength and flush old toxins out of the body with our 4-day *Short Home Cleanse*. (Chapter 12)

6. To strengthen digestion and ensure proper lymphatic drainage of every cell in the body, we must move our bodies. Finish the job of our digestive reboot and prevent further problems with my *Eat Wheat* Workout. (Chapter 13)

7. Finally, we all know it is our crazy minds that cause most of our stress and health concerns. Don't forget to address the impact our minds and emotions have on our digestive strength, overall health and happiness. (Chapter 14)

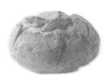

GROUND ZERO:
YOUR INTESTINAL SKIN

T he first step in rebuilding the digestive system is in knowing how to troubleshoot it. Understanding its logic will allow you to ask yourself some simple questions with regard to each aspect of the digestive process. While some people may need a total reboot of the digestion, many others can zero in on the weak link, restore that function, and then go about the business of digesting wheat and dairy once again.

Please use this book as a digestive rehab buffet, where you can help yourself to as much as you want from the array of digestive reset tips included. The key—and the goal—is to not only be able to digest hard-to-digest foods and avoid a restrictive diet, but to ensure that environmental toxins (remember, they even can be found on organically grown foods[38]) are properly digested and eliminated out of the body. *A healthy detoxification process cannot happen unless you are digesting well.*

Foods to Heal from the Inside Out

The lining of the intestines is made up of a type of epithelium or skin much like the skin on your body, just turned inside out. The health of the inner skin that lines the intestines will be reflected in the health, radiance and complexion of the skin on the outside. The intestinal skin is the first line of defense against stress, as all of our stress is processed through the intestinal wall. When the intestinal skin is overwhelmed by stress, undigested proteins, processed food chemicals and environmental toxins, it can break down and become inflamed. This can alter the health, function and quantity of the beneficial intestinal bacteria, break down digestion and assimilation of nutrients and let unwanted foods and toxins enter into the bloodstream and lymphatic system.

As you begin to repair and support the health of the intestinal skin and upper digestive system, it is best to avoid any foods that you are currently intolerant to, so your system can focus on healing and repairing. Once you have rebooted and strengthened your digestive function, you can slowly introduce non-toxic, non-processed versions of these foods.

When babies are born, they are fed breast milk until they start breaking teeth. Once their teeth start coming in, it is then time to start introducing "solid" foods, like applesauce, rice cereal, cooked bananas, and cooked, mashed vegetables. Traditionally, this was done very slowly in order to train the digestive system to handle these new foods. Cooking baby food and mixing it with a bit of water is a way of predigesting it, rendering it much easier for the baby to digest, especially during the initial test phase.

As adults, many of us have overeaten hard-to-digest, processed foods. As a result, we have stressed out our intestinal skin and microbes to a point where we have become intolerant to many foods.

For thousands of years, traditional cultures have been feeding their babies a well-cooked gruel made from watered-down rice and beans. In India, they created an Ayurvedic superfood that combines long grain rice and a bean called the split yellow mung bean. This mixture, called kitchari, was designed to soothe and nourish the intestinal skin. Today, in much of India, it is still the first food given to a baby and it is prescribed as a medicinal food and for convalescence for the elderly.

Before brown rice was de-husked and processed by machines to become white rice, parents would painstakingly take the time to remove the husk by hand from long grain rice. Then, they would hand-split the yellow mung beans to de-husk them as well, rendering the mung bean extremely easy to digest. This process would take days to make enough kitchari for their needs. They would then cook the rice and split yellow mung beans together for at least an hour with lots of water and spices to support digestion. In addition, they would add a small amount of ghee (clarified unsalted butter) to this mixture to help support the health of the intestinal tract. Remember, in Chapter 3, how we discussed that ghee is loaded with butyric acid, which is actually made in the intestinal tract by a variety of microbes to support gut health and immunity?[196, 197, 199] You will find the recipe for kitchari in Appendix C. Not only is it a great food for babies and the sick, but it's also a very nutritious, delicious, soothing and healing food for growing children, teenagers and adults.

Recently, there has been some impressive science supporting the benefits of the whole mung bean. Scientists have found that the 2 major mung bean flavonoids, vitexin and isovitexin, were able to turn off one of the body's major anti-aging switches called High Mobility Group Box 1 (HMGB1). HMGB1 triggers the release of toxic and degenerative cytokines in the body which can damage the intestinal wall.[381] In another study, mung bean flavonoids helped increase survival rates in animals from certain poisons by a whopping 82 percent.[382]

Known as the "anti-gas bean," mung beans were found to be virtually free of any "flatulence factors," suggesting that it may be the only bean that does not produce gas.[383] According to Ayurveda, it is the only bean classified as anti-vata or anti-gas. It is no surprise that Ayurveda chose this bean as the "intestinal repair bean" over all others.

Here are some of the other benefits of this amazing legume:

- It is packed with minerals including magnesium and phenols.[384]
- It has powerful antioxidant properties that support heart health.[385]
- It supports healthy blood sugar levels and reduces the damaging effects of glycation.[386]

- It produces the fatty-acid butyrate in the gut, thus supporting the health of the intestinal wall.[387, 388]
- It supports healthy weight loss and cravings by increasing the "I am full" hormone, cholecystokinin (CCK).[389]

You can eat kitchari as a staple in your diet as you start the repair process of your intestinal skin. For those who are concerned about eating rice, you can replace it with quinoa or millet. See the recipe for kitchari in Appendix C.

When we think of other foods that help support or help repair intestinal health, they would be well-cooked, since uncooked or raw vegetables would have too much indigestible fiber that can irritate the gut wall.

Some of my favorite "repair" foods are:
- Sweet potatoes
- Cooked beets
- Cooked apples
- Seeds, rather than nuts, which are harder to digest
- Well-cooked or steamed vegetables
- Oatmeal, rice, quinoa, millet
- Small, well-cooked beans or legumes (like mung beans) are easier to digest at first, compared to larger beans
- Healthy oils like ghee, coconut and olive oil
- Small amounts of well-cooked white meats or fish
- Small amounts of raw honey: 1–2 teaspoons per day
- Ginger, cinnamon, fennel and cardamom tea

Consider adding a small amount of organic fermented foods to each meal:
- Yogurt (Ideally without added sugar. Buy plain yogurt and add your own natural sweetener like maple syrup.)
- Kimchi
- Miso
- Tempeh

- Fermented vegetables
- Kombucha
- Olives
- Pickles

The Large Intestine

You can easily troubleshoot issues of the large intestine by becoming aware of the health and regularity of your bowel movements. The skin of the gut is like the three little bears. It has to be just right—not too dry and therefore constipating, and not too wet, as that can cause an excess of mucus production and loose stools or mucus in the stool. Healthy assimilation of nutrients, detoxification of toxins, and healthy microbes lining the intestines depend on a balanced environment of the intestinal skin.

A healthy bowel movement is a complete elimination, occurring within the first hour or so after waking up in the morning. It should be somewhat firm—not too hard and not too soft. The key is that it should feel like a complete and satisfying evacuation. It can be helped along with a large glass of water, or lemon water to start the day. However, if you need a cup of coffee, a bran muffin, a laxative (natural or otherwise), or some other ritual to get you to go, this is an indication that your digestive system is compromised and your intestinal skin needs attention.

What does this have to do with digesting wheat and dairy, which is mostly digested upstream, in the stomach and small intestine? The health of the intestinal skin, which is literally the skin that lines the intestinal tract, is a major factor in determining how efficiently waste will leave the body. If you tend towards constipation or loose stools, toxins can congest the lymphatic system that drains the intestines, as described in Chapter 4. Once the lymph is congested, toxic fats can be reabsorbed back to the liver and gallbladder where, over time, the upper digestion—responsible for breaking down wheat and dairy—will be compromised. Moreover, the health of the intestinal skin will determine the health of the body's intestinal microbes, which not only digest wheat and dairy, but are the foundation for all aspects of human health.[66]

Meet the Second Brain

The large intestine is where 90 percent of the trillions of microbes live in your body.[66] It is also the site where 95 percent of the serotonin in the body is manufactured and stored, allowing only 5 percent of the body's serotonin to be in the brain at any giving time.[390] The gut, which is now termed "the second brain," uses benefical microbes to manufacture many other brain chemicals, vitamins and enzymes that the body could not live without. According to Ayurveda, the large intestine is considered the seat of the entire nervous system, which means that the brain and the entire nervous system is regulated and governed by what happens in the gut.[239, 241, 245, 247, 250]

Stress—be it from mental, emotional, or physical, or from going against the circadian rhythms—is directly processed through the gut, not the brain. Lining the intestinal tract are trillions of microscopic microbes that do the heavy lifting for just about every physiological function of the body.[66]

Since we now know that these microbes determine our immunity, health, longevity, happiness, mood, and just about everything else, including the ability to digest wheat and dairy, we need to pay close attention to *their* well-being to support *our* well-being.[239, 240, 249, 391-395]

The villi and lacteals that line the intestinal wall are literally lined with microbes. These microbes are extremely sensitive to any stress we are under, any toxins we are exposed to, and the foods we eat.

The Bidirectional Gut-Brain Axis

By way of what is called the "gut-brain axis," stressors can alter the health of the microbiome, and the altered microbiome can send stress signals to the brain, which can alter mood, immunity, lymph flow, energy, joy and, you guessed it, the ability to digest wheat and dairy.[239, 240, 249, 391-397]

The brain takes its cue from the microbiome, then sends those messages to every cell of the body, which in turn speaks to the brain, all in a bidirectional flow of information between the gut and the brain.[398, 399] The gut microbiome is so powerful that, in one study, they found that greater microbial diversity was associated with more extraverted temperament in children.[252]

According to Ayurveda, the focus for intestinal health is on the repair of the intestinal skin rather than giving long-term herbal laxatives, digestive enzymes, or probiotics. In the intestinal tract, there are 3 general types of microbes: Good guys, bad guys, and spectators who do nothing but take up a lot of valuable intestinal real estate. In fact, studies suggest that, in the U.S., we have less healthy microbes than spectators and bad bugs.[73] We know that there are specific microbes responsible for the digestion of wheat and dairy, and we know that the microbiome in the U.S. is much less diverse that in other parts of the world.[73] It's no wonder we, as a culture, are having trouble digesting hard-to-digest foods.

How It All Works: A Quick Recap

I have now talked about how when gluten or casein go undigested in the upper digestion, not to mention deleterious effects of the pesticides sprayed on wheat crops.[62] These factors and more will act as intestinal irritants in the small and large intestines, dramatically altering their function.

We have also explored how, if the gluten and casein were properly broken down in the stomach and upper small intestine, much of the issues with gluten and dairy intolerances would be resolved. The problem is how poor digestion upstream in the stomach will affect the digestion downstream in the gut, and vice versa—they both have to be brought back into balance.

In addition, you have learned that when the gluten and casein make their way into the intestines, they will inflame the intestinal skin and separate and congest the villi and lacteals, allowing undigested proteins and toxins to enter into the lymphatic system and the bloodstream. This is where the hypersensitivity symptoms of wheat and dairy really do become a problem.

As a result of these hard-to-digest proteins irritating the intestinal skin, inflammatory toxic proteins like zonulin can be produced, which are linked to many wheat intolerance symptoms.[58]

You also now know that the lymph around the intestines is connected to lymph that is trying to drain the brain, the skin, the joints, the nervous system, the respiratory tract, the reproductive system, and yes, every cell of the body.[5, 10, 16, 203, 219, 221]

All of this makes weak digestion and broken-down intestinal skin a true crisis, but let's address the root cause of it rather than just focusing on the symptoms. This is a much bigger issue than the symptoms we may experience when eating wheat and dairy.

Why a Healthy Gut Matters

According to Ayurveda, the intestinal tract is a barrier that is designed to determine what foods—and even what toxins—are allowed to pass through and literally become "you." As far as the body goes, if something is still in the intestines, it has not become "you" yet, as the intestinal skin is still a functional barrier separating "you" from the outside world.

The intestinal microbes not only regulate the functions of the body, they also "feel" everything. They have been scientifically found to be affected by emotions and feelings[400] and pass information epigenetically to the genes found in every cell, in order to keep the genetic code informed of what's happening in the inner and outer worlds.[401-403]

For instance, a plant sprayed with a pesticide will likely suffer a genetic mutation—and this happens all the time—the mutation will be transferred or passed on to the microbes on the plant. And then, when we eat that plant, the mutated microbes pass this genetic information to the microbes in the gut, and then transferred to the genes inside of your body.[404-406] Healthy intestinal skin provides a barrier and only lets a certain amount of these mutations pass through. All of this is to be sure that the human genes are getting the required intelligence to survive and adapt in an ever-changing toxic world.

The intestinal skin is both a barrier to protect and inform the body of the changes and dangers of the outside world while delivering the needed nutrients to thrive. If the intestinal skin breaks down, there is a risk of too many mutations, toxins, glutens or casein proteins passing through the intestinal wall into the lymph, liver and bloodstream, predisposing the body to related chemical, allergenic, and hypersensitivity reactions.

Dry Intestinal Skin or Symptoms of Constipation

The first step in helping you digest wheat and dairy well is to help you repair the intestinal skin, and this will be reflected in a healthy, regular stool.

Stress can alter the microbiology of the intestinal skin and result in intestinal dryness or a form of constipation. There are a handful of remedies for constipation, but few do it without laxatives, which can lead to dependencies. The most common herbal laxatives—like senna or cascara sagrada—are bowel irritants that stimulate the bowels to contract.[407, 408] Over time, they can desensitize the bowels and eventually stop working. Even magnesium, which is thought to be a harmless laxative, works by pulling water out of the intestines to hydrate the stool. Long-term use can dehydrate the bowels and even demineralize the intestinal skin.

The key to resolving this problem is NOT to take laxatives, but to tone and lubricate the skin of intestines. The classic herb in Ayurveda to accomplish this is called triphala, which is a combination of 3 fruits:[409]

1. **Amalaki:** Helps repair the intestinal skin
2. **Bibhitaki:** Pulls excess mucus off the intestinal wall
3. **Haritaki:** Tones the muscles responsible for an actual bowel movement

These 3 fruits together support bowel tone, muscular function, and contractibility of the intestinal wall, strengthening peristalsis and thereby supporting smooth digestion, assimilation, and elimination. Triphala also helps maintain an appropriate balance of mucus lining, the skin of intestinal wall, preventing and clearing excess mucus buildup—which can hinder assimilation—and making sure a healthy layer of mucus remains, which soothes the digestive tract, supports healthy bacteria, and buffers against strong digestive acids.[410]

While triphala is not a laxative, it provides healthy elimination support. If the intestines are particularly dry or chronically constipated, I like to add demulcent or slimy herbs like slippery elm bark, marshmallow root, and licorice root to the triphala. This addition makes it much easier to wean off the triphala, which is always my goal—to become self-sufficient and not dependent on supplements.

Note: The bile that flows from the liver and gallbladder is the actual regulator of the stool and is often required to effectively treat constipation. I will discuss this further in Chapter 10.

Stools on the Loose

When the intestinal tract gets chronically irritated, the intestinal skin—which is lined with mucus membranes—can react by secreting excess mucus. This can cause loose stools or diarrhea. If the problem gets worse, the mucus can be produced in such quantities that you can begin to see mucus in your stool.

This is different from a bout of diarrhea when you are sick from a cold or food poisoning. This is a chronic condition where the excess mucus can bog down or even flatten the villi of the intestinal wall. When this happens, the ability to absorb nutrients and process toxins becomes compromised, and the environment for the proliferation of microbes that support the digestive process is affected.

The best herb I have found to naturally restore the health of the intestinal skin, intestinal discomfort, and reverse the tendency for loose stools is amalaki. Amalaki (*Emblica officinalis*), also known as Indian gooseberry, is a small fruit from the amla tree. Amalaki may be most well-known for its support of antioxidant activity and healthy skin via the encouragement of collagen and elastin production.[411-413] In this way, amalaki supports not only the health of the outer skin, but also the health and elasticity of the inner skin that lines the gut, respiratory tract, arteries, and all of the mucus membranes in the body.

Note: Other important herbs for the intestinal skin that I discuss in Chapter 10 are brahmi (Centella asiatica) and turmeric (Curcuma longa).

A Complete Digestive Overhaul

When there is mucus in the stool, the digestion is extremely delicate or sensitive, or the situation is chronic with bloating, gas, and abdominal pain, I tend to start from scratch in terms of rebooting the digestive system. This is a sign that the intestinal skin or mucus membranes of the entire digestive tract are irritated and producing reactive mucus. For this, I like to employ some first aid for the entire digestive tract.

My favorite therapy for this is a concentrated tea or decoction made out of chopped (not ground) slippery elm bark, licorice root, and marshmallow root that I have been using successfully in my practice for almost 30 years.

To antidote both the dryness and the overly damp mucous membranes, I have not found a better solution than this decoction, taken throughout the day for a month, to reset healthy intestinal and microbial function. Each of these herbs are naturally slimy and demulcent, which means that they will soften and soothe the dry and irritated mucous membranes all the way from the throat to the stomach to the small and large intestines. It is like coating the entire digestive tract with a protective mucilaginous, prebiotic, microbe-boosting Band-Aid for a month. During this time, new intestinal skin can grow, a healthy intestinal environment can be restored, and healthy microbes can repopulate.

 Tip: Amalaki, triphala, or a colonizing strain of probiotics, can be used here as needed for digestive repair, along with the slippery elm-licorice root-marshmallow root formulation.

When these 3 herbs are cooked down into a tea or concentrated decoction, the soluble fiber from their roots and barks are released. The soluble fiber is naturally slippery, and therefore offers soothing support to the dried-out intestinal mucosa.

The soluble fiber from these herbs also feeds the intestinal microbes and acts as a natural prebiotic for the microbiome.[414] This is a critical part of the tea's restorative effect—to create an environment that will allow the healthy microbes to proliferate while restoring the function and environment for the intestinal villi and gut mucosa to digest, detox, and assimilate nutrients optimally. Let's learn more about each of the ingredients in this demulcent concoction:

Licorice **(Glycyrrhiza glabra)**
- Licorice is a classic Ayurvedic herb used for thousands of years worldwide as a natural lubricant and demulcent for the intestinal and respiratory

airways. Licorice naturally lubricates and soothes mucus membranes and, as an adaptogen, it protects them from stress and environmental irritants and pollens.[415] Licorice quells the production of excess reactive mucus, and it supports the function of other herbs when taken conjunctly.[415] It is calming for an over-active nervous system, cooling the excess fire element in the body, and can liquefy and reduce extra mucus or congestion.

Slippery Elm Bark (Ulmus fulva)

- Slippery elm has long been used for digestive and intestinal concerns because of its demulcent, lubricating, and gut-protective properties.[416] Along with its mucilaginous, protective properties for the intestinal wall, it has been shown to support healthy antioxidant activity in the intestinal tract.[415]

- Like licorice, slippery elm has a sweet taste and cooling action. It balances an overactive nervous system and fiery constitution in the same way licorice does. As a result of its more mucilaginous properties, it creates a thick layer of protection that covers the entire intestinal tract.

Marshmallow Root (Althaea officinalis)

- Marshmallow Root is perhaps the most demulcent of the 3 herbs in this formula. It has been found to protect the stomach lining from excess acid and protect the intestinal tract from intestinal irritants, such as the toxic form of carrageenan or glyphosate.[417] Medicinally, it has been approved by the German Commission E (the German equivalent of the U.S. FDA) in supporting inflammation of the gastric mucosa, and for irritation of the oral and pharyngeal mucosa.[417]

- Like both licorice and slippery elm, marshmallow is a soluble fiber, which means it will be broken down by the stomach, but not absorbed. This allows it to offer the gut, where most of the microbes reside, a handsome feast of the fibers and nutrients these 3 herbs contain.

- Marshmallow is cooling for fiery constitutions, soothing and calming for anxious, overactive nervous systems and, as it is mucus-producing, it will increase congestion—a good thing in this instance—as we are trying to coat and protect the intestines from top to bottom over the course of 1 month of this therapy.

Make a Decoction or Tea At Home

The key to the success of this intestinal and microbial reset is to take these 3 herbs as a tea or concentrated decoction for a month or 2. If your intestinal tract is not in a severely inflamed condition, then you can use the tea. The tea tastes great and can be used as a maintenance beverage as well. You must source these herbs in a chopped—not ground—form. If you use ground herbs, you will make "mud" and it won't work. If you are concerned that your intestinal tract is in a reactive state and needs extra support, do your best to follow the decoction instructions.

⸺⟫⟫ Decoction Recipe ⟪⟪⸺

Ingredients:
- 1 tablespoon chopped licorice
- 1 tablespoon chopped slippery elm bark
- 1 tablespoon chopped marshmallow root
- 2 quarts water

Directions:
1. Soak 1 tablespoon of each of the chopped herbs—or 3 tablespoons of a pre-mixed, chopped mixture of all 3 herbs—in a boiling pot filled with 2 quarts of water overnight.
2. Soaking overnight is not mandatory, but it gives you a stronger decoction.
3. Boil the mixture down to 1/2 quart in the morning.
4. Strain the mixture through a metal strainer, using a large spoon to push it through.
5. Save the liquid and discard the herbs.
6. This should make 2 cups to sip on throughout the day.

---

7. Take 1 tablespoon of the liquid every 2 hours on an empty stomach for 1 month, and sometimes for 2 months if needed.

⨀⨀⨀ Tea Recipe ⨀⨀⨀

Ingredients:
- 1/3 tablespoon chopped licorice
- 1/3 tablespoon chopped slippery elm bark
- 1/3 tablespoon chopped marshmallow root
- 1 cup water

Directions:
1. To make tea, take equal amounts of the 3 herbs, totaling about 1 tablespoon altogether.
2. Steep this mixture in hot water until it becomes tea strength.
3. Drink 3–6 cups a day for 1–2 months, or as needed for maintenance.

Restore a Healthy Microbiome

With the discovery of the microbiome, which is the entire population of the body's microbes or bacteria, a new frontier in science and healthcare was born. Although it is still in its infancy, there is compelling evidence suggesting the numerous health benefits of taking probiotics. While the benefits of probiotics were once thought to be restricted to gut and digestive health, new research on the gut-brain axis is connecting our microbiome to the health of the brain, immunity, bone density, blood sugar, mood and even our intuition... and this is the short list.[418-420]

We should also realize that there is no magic bullet when it comes to probiotics. While there is plenty of science suggesting that they work well, the key is to establish an environment for a healthy and diverse microbiome to proliferate. This all starts with the health of the intestinal skin.

For example, if you flattened out all the villi and lacteals of the intestinal tract, it would cover the area of a studio apartment up to a tennis court.[421] Think for a minute how many people you could fit on a tennis court, and then imagine that your intestinal skin would cover the entire court. Then imagine an army of microscopic beneficial microbes blanketing the court as well—that's a lot of bugs!

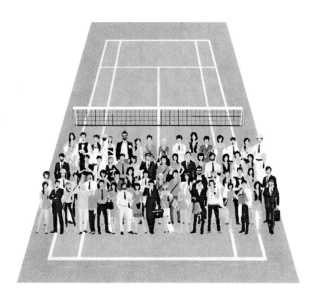

No doubt we have what seems like a ridiculous amount of intestinal surface area for a reason. These microbes manufacture hormones, vitamins, and neurotransmitters that help detox and assimilate nutrients while playing a role in almost every human bodily system.[66] Clearly, there are lots of backup villi in case of intestinal damage from stress, aging, toxins and potential infections. This is why most of the wheat and dairy intolerances take place insidiously over a very long period of time.

Transient Versus Colonizing Probiotics

To think we can just pop a probiotic to cure our digestive woes is giving ourselves false hope. Colonizing probiotics—while still very rare in the marketplace—actually adhere to the gut wall, become permanent residents, and build microbial diversity. Transient probiotics work well and support health in many ways, but once you stop them, the intestinal microbes tend to go back to the way they were. Unlike most transient probiotic products, which usually list the general strain of the microbe like lactobacillus or bifidobacterium, colonizing strains list the *exact* strain of the microbe that the research was done on.

For example, in one study, a specific strain of the colonizing probiotic called Bifidobacterium lactis HN019 was shown to adhere to the gut wall and increase microbial diversity in a study group of subjects over 60 years of age.[422-424] While the science studying our microbes is still in its infancy, it is clear that diversity matters, and westerners have significantly less microbial diversity than other cultures around the world.[422-424]

There are 3 specific strains of bugs that I have found as documented to adhere to the gut wall and colonize inside the gut.[420, 422-425] I highly recommend that a probiotic supplement contain some or all of these strains of colonizing microbes.

1. Lactobacillus acidophilus La-14[420, 425]
2. Lactobacillus plantarum Lp-115[420, 425]
3. Bifidobacterium lactis HN019[420, 422-425]

Even with the addition of a probiotic, it is still important to keep introducing more good bugs into your digestive tract through your diet. Do your best to add naturally lacto-fermented foods to at least 1 meal a day. Eat these as condiments, in very small amounts. A little goes a long way to create diverse strains and bacterial richness to your new temple of good bugs! New colonizing probiotic strains are being discovered as new research becomes available. Keep up with this emerging science by receiving my free video newsletter at LifeSpa.com.

Our Euro-Bug Study

I was so intrigued by the concept of colonizing probiotics that I decided to perform my own unpublished pilot study to confirm the results of the previous studies I cited above. We asked 10 Americans who were headed to Europe for a summer vacation for at least 2 weeks to be a part of our study. We gave half the group a combination of colonizing probiotics, while the other half of the group did not take a probiotic. We measured their microbiome 2 weeks before and 2 weeks after their trip.[426]

The results were profound. The group that took the probiotic had 60 percent more diverse microbes in their gut, compared to 33 percent increased diversity in the group that did not take a probiotic. All 10 participants saw an increase in their microbiome diversity after spending a couple of weeks in Europe, but the group that took the probiotics saw almost twice as much microbial diversity.[426]

If we can create a more suitable intestinal environment for more beneficial bacteria, and repopulate the gut with colonizing probiotics that will rebuild a healthy microbiome, this is a great step towards digestive health and self-sufficiency without taking lifelong probiotics.

Grow New Bugs
The following is a 2-step comprehensive plan for restoring gut health:

1. Support the intestinal mucus membranes by bringing the elimination back into balance with either triphala, amalaki, or the prebiotic, soluble fiber tea made from the slippery elm, licorice root, and marshmallow root mixture to create the best possible environment for healthy microbes to thrive.
2. Introduce healthy, *colonizing* probiotics for a few months—instead of the rest of your life with transient probiotics—to help establish new beneficial, permanent bacterial residents to proliferate in your gut and enhance your health and digestion.

Note: If there is an overgrowth of undesirable bacteria in the small and large intestines, I have great clinical success adding a beneficial yeast called Saccharomyces boulardii, which has been shown to knock out undesirable yeast and bacteria in the digestive tract. More on this in Chapter 11.

Thinking and Feeling Microbes

Researchers now theorize that when an individual is under stress, certain stress-related chemicals are produced in the gut. These stress chemicals alter the microbiome of the gut and disturb digestion, immunity and the production of mood-supporting neurotransmitters.[402] For example, changing one's mood can be as simple as changing your good bacteria. When fearful mice had a fecal transplant with aggressive mice, the fearful mice became aggressive.[427]

At the University of Wisconsin, researchers found that pregnant mice that were repeatedly startled and stressed during their pregnancies had babies who had significantly less lactobacilli and bifidobacteria (good microbes) in their guts.[402]

A 2010 study published in *Brain, Behavior, and Immunity* observed mice that were forced to live with a social disrupter—a mouse that was very aggressive and disruptive. Living with such a mouse changed the bacteria in the guts of the healthy normal mice. Their good bacteria were decreased, the bad bacteria proliferated, and the mice experienced numerous compromised health and immunity-related conditions.[222]

Why do these studies matter to the digestion? The state of our digestion is inextricably tied to the state of our brain, our mood, and our well-being, and vice versa.[428] Thus, with healthy digestion, our mood and sense of well-being improves, the health of our microbiome improves and thus, so does our digestion.[222, 249, 250, 393, 396, 398, 399, 402, 420, 427-438]

Don't Hurt Your (Gut) Feelings

Taking time to sit down, relax, dine, and digest your food are much-revered, well-studied, health-promoting practices.[439] There are even well-studied benefits of taking a short rest or "siesta" after the meal to help the body efficiently digest a meal.[440] Furthermore, Ayurvedic texts state that lying on your left side or resting after a meal will boost digestive strength and ward off an after-the-big-meal crash by allowing the food to be properly digested and released from the stomach naturally. Modern science supports these ancient principles,[440-442] suggesting that taking time to relax and eat,[439] taking rest after the meal,[440] and/or taking a walk after the meal[443]—all traditional Ayurvedic techniques—will help to strengthen digestion, support weight loss, and balance blood sugar levels after meals.

Modern research indicates that emotional stress will alter the health of the intestinal skin and the function of the microbiome, which is intimately involved in digestion. To take advantage of the research—like how a restful, relaxed environment during meals is beneficial for our health and digestion[439, 443]—follow another ancient Ayurvedic saying: "Better not to eat, than eat while angry." Make your meals a scheduled, relaxed event that you look forward to. And then, once at the table, take some time to relax and then begin to eat your food.

Ayurveda takes this concept even further with another old saying that is now backed by science: "What you see, you become." This means that whatever you choose to give your attention to will shape you, and thereby become you. Feelings and beliefs make up much of what we give our attention to, altering the microbes of the gut.[400] When the microbes in our gut are impacted by stress hormones, it has a significant impact on our health, and ultimately our digestion.[222]

Consider these 3 mindsets:

- **Love-Joy** is a state of mind that is fully content within itself. It does not require anything from the outside to make it happy.
- **Fight-or-Flight** is a state of mind that requires stimulation to be happy. Satisfaction comes from the stimulation of our senses from the outside world.
- **Protection** is a state of mind that has become overstimulated, exhausted, and depleted. It is inward, depressed and withdrawn.

The "fight-or-flight" and "protection" qualities trigger a sympathetic nervous system response that literally shuts off the digestive process, while the "love-joy" mindset activates the parasympathetic nervous system that turns on and strengthens the digestive process. The "fight-or-flight" and "protection" mindsets can put stress on your emotions and your microbes,[400] and cause imbalances in your microbiome, contributing to difficulties digesting hard-to-digest foods. Our microbes are extremely sensitive, and thrive in a healthy, balanced, peaceful, loving environment.[222, 444-448]

While all of us have experienced all 3 of the above mindsets, only acts of love and relaxation turn on digestive strength, have a positive effect on the microbiology, give a life-supporting epigenetic effect, actually lengthen chromosomal telomeres, thereby helping to curb the aging process, and have a direct effect on the genetic code.[401, 403, 444-449]

Don't miss out on the most simple and potentially most profound therapy to boost digestive strength—sit, relax, dine. Take time to enjoy each and every meal.

Looking Ahead

Now that we have discussed how to heal the gut, join me as we proceed to Chapter 9 and talk about healing the lymph—the primary source of food allergy symptoms.

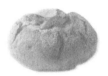

Chapter 9
LYMPH RX

R emember Mary, who had many of the symptoms associated with gluten and dairy intolerances and how we were able to link her symptoms to congested lymph issues? Her chronic lymphatic congestion was directly linked to her food sensitivities, rashes, migraines, achiness and moodiness. Once we were able to remove the stagnation from her lymph, the litany of health concerns she had carried for years began to finally resolve. In this chapter, I want to share the lymph therapies that I used with Mary that are often required to eradicate the symptoms of wheat and dairy intolerance.

As you may recall, the lymphatic system starts inside the intestinal tract as lacteals within small finger-like projections called villi, whose function depends on the health and environment of the intestinal skin.

The intestinal skin and lymph are designed so that large proteins and fats are pulled off the intestinal tract into the lymphatic system, where they are processed by the immune system and lymph nodes that line the lymphatic system. Large, undigested proteins like casein and gluten, as well as fat-soluble environmental pollutants and toxins can also be pulled into the lymphatic system, like we saw with Mary.

If your lymphatic system is overwhelmed with large proteins (say, from gluten) and fat-soluble toxins, the lymph will congest and your immune system can become hypersensitive and overreact. This overreaction, or overzealous immune response, can result in something as simple as an allergy or something as complex as an autoimmune condition. In between these two extremes, we see a host of possible symptoms associated with lymphatic congestion as a result of improper digestion and the absorption of toxins into the lymphatic system. Lymphatic congestion can also back up the lymph flow from the brain. This congestion has been scientifically linked to inflammation, auto-immunity, depression and mood alterations.[5-9]

Classic lymphatic-related symptoms are joint pain, swelling, hives, eczema, inflammation, headaches, brain fog, stiffness in the morning, achiness, gas, bloating, digestive discomfort, anxiety, depression and chronic fatigue. Mary experienced almost all of these lymph-related concerns.

Stress and Lifestyle Affect your Lymph

Everyone's physiology is unique; we are all born with a unique blueprint, with its strengths and weaknesses. On top of that, our home, family and society contribute their influences that either further strengthen or weaken the digestion and the lymphatic system. It's important to take some time and reflect upon what internal *and* external stressors you have been influenced by, and contemplate when these began—perhaps it was even stressors from in utero or childhood.

How you are digesting your food may be intricately connected to how you are digesting your life experiences and vice versa. In Chapter 14, entitled "Mind over Batter," I will discuss these concepts further.

There is also new science that suggests our DNA has many switches attached to chromosomes, and they are either switched on or off.[450] Researchers are now finding that these switches can be flipped on or off during our lifetime based on stress, as well as behavioral and environmental influences.[451] So it's important to be mindful of your lifestyle choices, as they are actually directly impacting your health and the way you digest.

Antioxidants, Aging, and Intestinal Lymph

The lymphatic system is a primary site for free radical damage, degenerative diseases, and accelerated aging. In addition to the blood, antioxidants like vitamin C, selenium, blueberries, pomegranates, and the long list of food-based antioxidants worked their anti-aging magic in the lymphatic system.

Groundbreaking research has linked accelerated aging to the breakdown of lymphatic vessels of the body. In particular, the lymphatic vessels that were linked to the degeneration and aging of the body were the mesenteric lymphatics, which line the intestinal tract. These lymphatic vessels are responsible for the lion's share of the body's immunity and are now shown to determine the speed in which we age.[452]

Both the gut-associated lymph on the outside of the large intestine and the mesenteric lymph that lines the small intestine is very vulnerable to toxicity. These lymphatics are also sensitive to stressors from inside the intestinal tract, which can express through conditions such as leaky gut or irritable bowel syndrome.

In this chapter, I will discuss the role of many lymph-movers and cleansers— antioxidant foods and herbs that will support optimal function of the lymphatic vessels lining the intestinal tract.

Rehydration Therapy

Rehydration Therapy Part 1

Let's discuss the importance of hydration. Lymph congestion has been linked to states of dehydration and a host of gastrointestinal issues, including inflammatory bowel syndrome. Science is pointing to the congestion of intestinal lymphatic vessels that predispose the body to intestinal irritation and inflammation.[215, 254]

About 2/3 of the population are dehydrated, and the lymphatic system seems to be most affected by proper hydration levels.[254] This is because the flow of fluid from inside the cell to outside the cell and into the lymphatic system *all* depends on osmotic pressures that are based on proper hydration.

The first lymphatic therapy technique is what I like to call "Hot Sips." To accomplish this, boil purified water and carry a thermos throughout the day, drinking 2–3 sips of the plain hot water every 10–15 minutes throughout the day. Continue this for about 2 weeks. Once in a while, you can squeeze a little lemon into this water. You can still drink other beverages such as tea and juice. During the day, just make a point of sipping hot water as much as possible.

This is an Ayurvedic cleansing therapy that has been used for thousands of years to help improve lymphatic function and help the body detoxify. Sipping hot water has a vasodilation effect that helps to increase the circulation and the ability for the lymphatic lacteals to function. Hot water is said to help detoxify the body better, and in the same way you would use hot water to clean a pot or dish, cold water simply does not have the same effect. In addition, hot water seems to increase the molecular activity in and around the cells that have come in contact with it. It is said that if you were to pour cold water onto dehydrated leather, the water would simply run off of it. If you were to pour hot water onto dehydrated leather, it would soften, hydrate and clean the leather. I have used the Hot Sips therapy clinically for more than 30 years and still use it today because of its great effectiveness.

I always tell my patients to simply try this technique for 1 day. If you do not find yourself craving this hot water at the end of the day, you are likely not dehydrated. Most people find themselves craving the hot water. Of course it sounds terribly boring, but you would be amazed at how good it tastes and how good you feel when you start this rehydration therapy. Remember to use good quality, filtered and purified water.

Hot Sips Science

In one study, sipping hot water was compared to cold water, and they found that hot water increases the speed in which the mucus passes through the respiratory tract. The cilia that line the respiratory tract contract about 20 times per second, and there are at least 200 of them per cell. It is the cilia's job to keep impurities from infecting the lungs. With hot water sips, the cilia transport impurities up from the bronchioles and sinuses more quickly, to be either coughed up and out of the body or swallowed. Smaller toxins or bacteria that slip through the cracks of the cilia are picked up by the lymph that line the respiratory tract and are carried to lymph nodes to be purified. The hot water may also dilate the upper respiratory lining and support the efficiency of the lymph drainage there as well. The conclusion was that sipping hot water may be an effective tool to manage upper respiratory infections.[453]

Sipping hot water compared to cold water also helped folks with indigestion and difficulty swallowing as a result of slow esophageal contractions. If you suffer from indigestion or have difficulty swallowing and usually drink an iced beverage with your meal, you might consider switching from drinking cold water to hot water, herbal tea or even try room temperature water instead.[454]

Rehydration Therapy Part 2
The second part of the Rehydration Therapy called your "Daily Ounces" is to drink 1/2 of your ideal body weight in ounces of water each day for the 2-week period of time. The hot water that you drink counts toward your ounces of water (room temperature is best) that you drink each day. This formula usually puts you a little higher than the recommended 6–8 glasses of water per day. It is important during a lymphatic therapy to keep the body well-hydrated.

Rehydration Therapy Part 3
The final aspect of Rehydration Therapy is to rehydrate the lining of the stomach. One of the most common causes of tummy aches for children is that they are dehydrated. The stomach is lined with a bicarbonate layer that is designed to buffer the acids in the stomach. This bicarbonate layer is 95 percent water by weight.[455] If the body and stomach are dehydrated, the stomach will simply not produce the acid required to break down and digest hard-to-digest foods like gluten and casein, as well as other hard-to-digest proteins.

This technique requires drinking about 12 ounces of room temperature water 15–30 minutes before eating a meal, which counts toward your Daily Ounces. This will allow the water to flood and then hydrate the buffer layer of the stomach. Then, when you start eating your meal, the stomach is prehydrated and completely willing to produce the needed acid required to digest just about anything. In one study, mentioned in Chapter 6, this technique was shown to improve digestion and increase weight loss and body mass index, simply by drinking water half an hour before you eat your meal.[323]

This technique is not to be confused with drinking copious amounts of water right before or with the meal. If you drink too much water either with the meal or right before the meal, you run the risk of diluting your stomach acid and actually weakening your digestive strength. The idea with regard to water before or with the meal is to drink just enough to create a soup-like consistency of the food inside the stomach. Again, much like the three little bears, it shouldn't be too much and it shouldn't be too little—the amount of water you drink has to be just right.

Rehydration Therapy is one of the most simple and profound ways to increase your digestive strength. It's quite amazing how water can increase the production of your stomach acid, help break down hard-to-digest proteins in wheat and dairy and, in turn, stimulate the production of bile in the liver and digestive enzymes in the pancreas and duodenum. It is a requirement that all of these functions be coordinated, so that the proper digestive microbiology can flourish, wheat and dairy can be digested properly, and environmental toxins and pollutants can be broken down that would otherwise find their way into our blood, fat, lymph, and brain.[23-27]

Lymph-Moving Foods from Season to Season

Plants that were historically used as dyes—such as berries, cherries, beets, saffron and turmeric—were commonly used to stimulate the lymph, and are loaded with antioxidants. Blueberries,[456] raspberries,[457] and strawberries[458] are all traditional dyes and well-documented antioxidants that support lymph function. The general rule of thumb is that if the food stains your fingers while eating it, it is likely a lymph-mover.

Spring: March through June

- Year-round, nature is providing foods that support lymph flow. In the spring, we see cherries, berries, and leafy greens harvested in abundance to support a natural spring cleaning in our bodies. The fluorescent green that consumes most landscapes in the spring reflects greens rich in chlorophyll. Chlorophyll is a powerful mover of the body's lymph.

Chlorophyll-rich spring greens are also required to repopulate the gut with a fresh source of beneficial microbes that impact most of the body's functions.[66]

• These spring foods are predominately alkaline, which also supports the lymph flow of the body. Root veggies and herbs like turmeric (*Curcuma longa*), red root (*Ceanothus americanus*), manjistha root (*Rubia cordifolia*), dandelion (*Taraxacum officinale*), nettles (*Urticaria dioica*), cleavers (*Galium aparine*), astragalus (*Astragalus membranaceus*) and others, are all spring-harvested and are powerful cleansing herbs for the lymph. Red root, for instance, has been traditionally used by native people to support healthy lymph flow and to help reduce inflammation and swollen glands.[459] Spring is the best season to alkalize the body with seasonal greens, and choosing alkaline foods during this season makes perfect sense.

Summer: July through October

• In the summer, there are more leafy greens and a variety of lymph-moving green veggies that are documented to increase lymphatic flow. Citrus fruits are loaded with vitamin C and flavonoids that support the integrity of the lymph vessels.[460] Other summer harvest fruits like apples, berries, cherries, grape skin and seeds, are loaded with lymph-moving procyanidins.[461]

Fall and Winter: November through February

• In the fall, nature's lymph-moving bounty includes pomegranates, beets, and cranberries, as well as another harvest of turmeric, dandelion, red root, and manjistha, queen's root (*Stillingia sylvatica*) and ocotillo (*Fouquieria splendens*) for a final lymph flush before winter. Spices like ginger, cinnamon, cardamom, coriander, and black pepper are all great lymph-movers as well, as are seeds of flax and chia—but my favorite lymph-moving seed is fennel. These fall foods sustain us into winter, when nature's growing season is mostly dormant because of the cold weather.

More Lymph-Moving Foods

Eating fennel and drinking tea made from fennel seeds and nettle are traditional ways to move the lymph. As a tea, fennel is effective for gas and bloating, and also supports the function of the intestinal lacteals, which help absorb nutrients—and particularly fats.[462] Fennel has also been shown to increase the white blood cells in the lymphatic system, thus supporting healthy immune function, and has been shown to be a powerful antioxidant and free-radical scavenger as well as an antimicrobial agent, protecting the gut against the proliferation of harmful bacteria and fungi.[462]

As I already mentioned, green leafy vegetables are highly alkaline, which support lymphatic drainage. A study in the journal *Nature Immunology* measured the effect of the *proteins* in leafy greens and cruciferous veggies on the innate lymphoid cells of the digestive tract, and found that they encouraged healthy lymphatic movement.[463] (This is of note, because most people don't usually think of green veggies for the importance of their proteins.) Innate lymphoid cells (ILC) are the immune-boosting cells that line the digestive tract and are responsible for protecting the body from allowing "bad" bacteria to proliferate. ILCs also help prevent undigested foods and toxins like gluten from passing through the intestinal wall into the lymphatic system.

These lymph cells that line the entire digestive tract are also believed to play an important role in controlling food hypersensitivities, unwanted weight gain, internal swelling, and the unhealthy proliferation of cells in the gut, so eat those greens![463]

An Apple (and Beet) a Day

As I mentioned before, apples as well as other lymph-moving antioxidant-rich fruits like berries, cherries, cranberries, grape skins and seeds, and pomegranates are high in procyanidins. In one study, apple procyanidins were found to reduce or prevent immune disorders such as allergies and autoimmune diseases through the lymphatic system.[461]

Beets are a powerhouse of anti-inflammatory, antioxidant-laden, liver-protective and anti-cancer agents that support healthy lymphatic function.[452, 464]

The combination of apples and beets make a great lymph-moving treat. These two, as we will see in the next chapter, are also my favorite bile-movers and bile-decongestants.

Enjoy this simple family favorite recipe of ours (kids love it!):

⁓ Apple-Beet Salad Recipe ⁓

Ingredients:
- 1 organic red beet
- 1 organic apple
- Juice of 1/2 lemon

Directions:
1. Wash, peel and grate 1 organic red beet
2. Wash and grate 1 organic apple
3. Add the juice of 1/2 organic lemon
4. Toss thoroughly
5. Enjoy!

Lymph-Moving Herbs

Manjistha (Rubia cordifolia)
- Perhaps Ayurveda's premier herbal lymphatic support is a root called manjistha (*Rubia cordifolia*, meaning "red root"). Classically used as a red dye, like its lymph-moving cousins mentioned above, manjistha is an herb I have been using clinically with great effectiveness for more than 30 years.
- In one study, manjistha was found to provide powerful liver support when the liver was exposed to higher levels of toxic chemicals. One mechanism by which manjistha was shown to do this was through boosting the production of glutathione levels. Glutathione is perhaps the body's most powerful antioxidant.[465]

- In two other studies, manjistha was found to be a potent antioxidant, and in one study it even out-performed some classic antioxidants, including vitamin E.[465, 466] Remember, antioxidants generally work their health-enhancing magic within the lymphatic system. Manjistha has also been shown to protect the good fats in the liver and lymph from lipid peroxidation, which is when good fats become bad fats within the body.[465]

Turmeric (**Curcuma longa**)

- Turmeric, which is a well-known cooking spice, possesses an important but less well-known quality of lymphatic flow support, and has been shown to markedly reduce swollen lymph glands.[467]
- Turmeric also supports healthy lymph flow and has been found to significantly decrease the risk of cancer-related metastasis. The lymphatic system is the body's highway for the immune system, and as we now know, many of the symptoms of gluten and dairy intolerance are simply due to congested lymph flow and an immune system stuck in traffic.[468]
- Turmeric also has been shown to increase bile flow from the liver and gallbladder, as well as maintain the integrity of the bile ducts that transport bile from the liver and gallbladder to the intestines, thus supporting our digestive ability.[469] See Chapter 10 for more in-depth coverage of turmeric. Turmeric also supports healthy intestinal skin.

Brahmi (**Centella asiatica**)

- Brahmi, otherwise known as *Centella asiatica* or gotu kola, is perhaps one of the most unique herbs for supporting healthy lymph flow and microcirculation as related to the classic signs of gluten and dairy intolerance. Most well-known for its support of cognitive function, new research has discovered lymph vessels that drain toxins from the brain that may explain why this herb is so useful for the brain fog and cognitive issues related to wheat and dairy.[5]

- Brahmi supports the health and repair of the skin cells that line the veins, lymph vessels and stomach, meaning not only is it helpful for balancing cellulite-related issues, it also supports healthy circulation of the blood and lymph, and healthy digestion to boot.[470, 471]

- Did you know that brahmi was traditionally used to increase the circulation of the brain? Now with the research pointing to the myriad ways it supports lymph drainage, cognitive benefits, and even the health of the skin of the stomach, it looks like it would be a great choice to boost digestive strength and resolve lymph-related symptoms that are so common in wheat and dairy intolerances.[5, 470, 471]

Tip: Brahmi is also a powerful herb for the skin, on both the outside and inside of the body; most importantly, the intestinal skin.

A Surprising Lymph-Mover

When I did my Ayurvedic training in India, we used to peel the white pith from oranges and pomegranates and dry and grind them. It was used as an Ayurvedic medicine for blood pressure. Healthy blood pressure depends greatly on good microcirculation and lymphatic drainage, or else pressure in the arteries can build up.

New research is showing that a flavonoid called *diosmin*—found in the pith or white part of the peel of certain citrus fruits like oranges—has a strong effect on moving and decongesting the lymphatic system. In fact, diosmin seems to affect all the circulatory drains of the body, supporting the healthy function, strength, and competence of the lymph, capillary and venous systems, and perhaps most notably affecting cellulite levels.[460]

Diosmin has been shown to support and prolong healthy venous tone when impacted by stress chemicals such as adrenaline or epinephrine,[472] as well as support the circulatory system's antioxidant systems.[473-476] Further, placebo-controlled human trials support the use of diosmin for the maintenance of healthy metabolism, microcirculation, fluid balance on a cellular level and lymph system function, which are all linked to congestive conditions such as cellulite and many of the concerns related to food intolerances.[477-481] With all these great health benefits, now there's even more reason to eat your citrus—to support lymphatic health!

 Tip: These lymph-moving herbs can be taken after meals, 3 times a day. The standard dose is 500mg or 1 standard "0"-size capsule.

Apple Cider Vinegar (ACV)

Apple cider vinegar—often called "sour wine"—is created by a natural lactic bacteria fermentation process. When allowed to ferment naturally, as in most natural store-bought ACV, it is rich in acetic acid, yeast, and other beneficial bacteria that support our health and well-being. It is a classic pre-meal drink to increase the stomach's HCl production and a great way to boost digestive fire. (More on this in Chapter 10.)

As a lymphatic tonic, ACV has been shown to stop the oxidation of fats and cholesterol in the body, as well as function as a powerful antioxidant for the lymphatic system.[482] In one study, mice were fed a high-cholesterol diet, and the mice that took apple cider vinegar saw greater levels of blood and lymphatic antioxidants like vitamins A and C, as well as glutathione and other free radical scavenging agents. Other studies suggest it is useful for lowering blood sugar, beneficial for the heart, reduces infections and protects the gut wall from tumor formation.[483]

Add up to 1 tablespoon of raw, unfiltered, organic apple cider vinegar to a large 12 ounce glass of water 15–30 minutes before meals for best results. It will boost stomach acid production and bile flow while supporting the protection of the intestinal wall and better lymphatic circulation. Make sure you buy organic apple cider vinegar with the "mother," which is a combination of natural yeast and acetic acid bacteria that have much to do with its medicinal properties.[483] Braggs is one national brand of unfiltered organic apple cider vinegar we can recommend.

Many folks find that when they take ACV before a meal, they tolerate gluten better. And if they are feeling the effects of a gluten reaction, many report that ACV is a great remedy for those symptoms. Once again, an ounce of ancient wisdom with a pound of science makes a pretty awesome remedy.

Alkaline Versus Acidic Foods

The intent of nature was for us to eat more of the foods that are in season, as I described in Chapter 6. When there are obvious symptoms of lymph congestion related to the poor and incomplete digesting of wheat and dairy, emphasizing more of the alkaline foods on the list below, in conjunction with seasonal eating, is imperative. Eating more alkaline foods is scientifically linked to a reduction in inflammation, the boosting of immunity, increased energy, balanced digestion, and balanced weight.[484-486]

A good goal to strive for is to eat a diet that is 2/3 alkaline, based on nature's changing bounty. The majority of alkaline foods are harvested in the spring and summer, while the acidic foods—more commonly the brown foods—are typically harvested in the fall for winter eating. Acidic foods warm the body and help rebuild and store some fat during the winter months. To accommodate the natural ebb and flow of seasonal foods and their respective microbiology, emphasize the alkaline list of foods in the spring and summer and the acidic food list in the winter.

While most experts agree we should all be eating a diet of 2/3 alkaline foods, this may be a difficult task for many people. As we heal and repair the intestinal skin and strengthen the upper digestion, it will become easier to be satisfied on lighter, more seasonal alkaline foods. In addition to the list below, please modify your seasonal food choices based on the seasonal grocery lists found in Appendix A.

ALKALINE FOODS Lymph-movers		ACIDIC FOODS Potential Lymph-congestors
VEGETABLES	**FRUIT**	**MISC**
Alfalfa sprouts	Apples	Alcohol
Beets & greens	Apricots, fresh & dried	Aspirin
Broccoli	Avocado	Chocolate
Brussel sprouts	Bananas	Coffee
Cabbage	Blackberries	Eggs and dairy
Carrots	Blueberries	Honey

Cauliflower	Cherries	Niacin
Celery	Dates	Mustard
Collard greens	Figs, fresh & dried	Pepper, black
Corn, fresh	Grapefruit	Meat, all
Cucumbers	Grapes	Nuts, all
Dulse	Lemons	Seeds
Green beans	Lychee nuts	Soft drinks
Green limas	Limes	Tea, black
Green peas	Mangoes	Vinegar - distilled
Green soy beans	Oranges	**BEANS**
Kale	Pineapple	Chickpeas
Kelp	Nectarines	Legumes
Leaf lettuce	Peaches	Lentils
Mushrooms	Pears	Soy, Tofu, Tempeh
Mustard greens	Raisins	**GRAINS**
Okra	Raspberries	Barley
Onions	**MISC**	Bread
Parsley	Lima beans	Cake
Peppers	Millet	Cereals, all
Potatoes	Cider	Corn flour
Parsnips	Maple syrup	Corn starch
Radishes	Molasses	Grains, except millet
Rhubarb		Oatmeal
Sauerkraut		Pasta
Spinach		Rice
Squash		Soda crackers
Turnip greens		Wheat bran
Tomatoes		Wheat germ
Watercress		Wheat products
Yams		**FRUIT**
		Cranberries
		Plums & prunes
		Fruits - canned

Seasonal Lymph Detox

Every spring and fall, nature delivers foods that naturally support a healthy detoxification. In the spring, lymph-movers and antioxidant-rich foods like bitter roots, leafy greens, and some berries and cherries are harvested. These spring foods force the body into a natural fat-burning state and instigate a natural, timely detox. The spring harvest is naturally low in fat, which forces the body to burn its own fat. Since the body is inclined to store fat-soluble toxins from chemicals, preservatives, and the environment in our fat,[23-27] the spring harvest presents the very best time for such a detox.

In the fall, at the end of summer, the body has accumulated an excess of summer's heat and nature has designed a seasonal detox to help the body dissipate any excess seasonal heat. Antioxidant-rich berries and fruits are in season, as are root veggies like turmeric, dandelion, ginger, and others. Apples, pomegranates, and watermelons are all extremely cooling foods, as well as blood- and lymph-cleansing, making them the perfect seasonal antidotes to the accumulation of the end-of-summer heat.

In nature, if the heat is not dissipated from the body, it will turn into dryness. Come winter, the cold temperatures help offset the heat, but any dryness left over from un-dissipated summer heat is only exacerbated by the innate dryness of winter. Excessive dryness in the winter can cause the respiratory mucus membranes to dry out, and if neglected, the mucus membranes will compensate by producing excess reactive mucus. Both dry mucus membranes and excessive reactive mucus can compromise immunity, congest the respiratory lymph, and predispose the body to bouts of the cold and flu.

Eating as close as possible to the seasonal harvest offers natural protection from the ebb and flow of nature's seasonal shifts, plus delivers seasonal microbes that help connect us to nature. The spring and fall are great times to help the body detoxify the lymph and liver with a home cleanse. Because of the sedentary nature of our modern culture, it is more important than ever to help support this seasonal cleansing process whenever possible. See Chapter 12 for instructions on how to perform a 4-day, self-guided, seasonal lymphatic and liver detox with a digestive reset at home.

Exercise Your Brain Drain

Perhaps the most effective lymph-mover is exercise. An abundance of research tells us that the lymphatic system—which transports the immune system, processes toxins and delivers nutrients—moves primarily when we sleep,[5] and when we move and exercise.[487, 488] It is becoming clearer that toxins drain from the brain and central nervous system in the spine through tiny lymph vessels when we sleep.[5] Yes, these lymph vessels are very small, which is why they have only recently been discovered, but that does not mean they are not important. In fact, they may be more important than ever thought.

These brain drain lymphatic channels, called glymphatics, have been found to drain up to 3 pounds of toxins like beta-amyloid plaque and other toxins from the brain each year. This is the equivalent of the entire weight of the brain in toxic waste every year.[5, 489]

When you combine the fact that the majority of humans are very sedentary compared to our hunter-gatherer ancestors who walked some 6–9 miles per day, according to Harvard professor Daniel Lieberman, author of *The Story of the Human Body*,[257] modern humans are not getting adequate activity during the day to support the needed lymph movement for optimal health.

Even in the last 50 years, activities such as washing clothes, dishes, and numerous other physical activities have become automated. We, as a culture, have been moving less and less, and this trend towards less activity has only been compounded in our current informational computer age, where millions of people spend hours each day sitting perfectly still in front of a screen of some kind.

As a result, there have been less lymph-moving muscular contractions and physical activity going on, and our natural removal of toxins via the major lymph channels has been severely compromised. Our daily exercise-induced toxin and lymph detoxification then falls upon the micro-toxin lymph drainage that takes place during our sleep—and to compound matters, many of us are not getting adequate amounts of sleep.

These microscopic lymph vessels that drain the brain and nervous system while we sleep are not designed or qualified to keep up with the demands of our modern, sedentary lifestyle. The sleep cycle of lymph drainage was meant to detox toxins from the brain, not the body.

These microscopic lymph channels can easily become overwhelmed, and new studies have linked autoimmune conditions, inflammation, anxiety, depression, and many of the symptoms related to gluten sensitivities to the congestion of these microscopic lymphatic vessels.[5-9]

It is interesting to note that the largest circulatory system of the body, and the one that is emerging as the most important—the lymph[16]—pumps primarily via muscular contraction and exercise. This is one of the reasons that exercise supports cardiovascular health.[490] Exercise has been shown to increase lymph drainage from the legs by 83 percent, suggesting that the key to taking the toxic stress off the lymphatic system is to exercise.[491]

Movement, exercise,[487, 488] and deep sleep[5]—all of which our modern culture has trouble with—are the major lymph movers of the body, and almost all of the gluten-related symptoms can be traced back to weak digestion, resulting in lymph congestion. Lymphatic fluid is not pumped from the heart like blood in the arteries and veins. Because the lymph drains back to the heart from the fingers and toes, flowing opposite the downward force of gravity, exercises that incorporate jumping are excellent for the lymph.

Lymph Tip: Jumping on a trampoline or mini-trampoline for just 10 minutes a day can have a profound effect on the lymph. Inverted yoga postures or anti-gravity hanging devices are also very effective for lymph flow.

The founder of Iyengar yoga, B.K.S. Iyengar, who lived vibrantly into his 90s, said that if he could boil all his success down to one yoga pose, it would be the headstand.[492] Curiously, it is one of the most effective lymph-moving yoga postures, as are all the inverted yoga postures—forward bend, legs-up-the-wall, or other safe inverted postures can be effectively used for lymph-moving benefits. My favorite series of yoga postures that move lymph while boosting digestive strength is Surya Namaskara, or the Sun Salutation. I describe its profound benefits in Chapter 13, and you can find Sun Salutation instructions, with optional modifications designed for everybody, in Appendix D.

There is much more to discuss regarding exercise, the lymph, and how proper exercise can help reset your digestive strength. This is such an important topic that I have dedicated Chapter 13, "The *Eat Wheat* Workout," to this topic.

Lymph Rx Review

Let's recap all of the ways that we can support healthy lymphatic flow for optimal health and digestion.

Rehydration Therapy

- Sip 2–3 sips of hot water every day for 2 weeks, every 10–15 minutes.
- Drink half of your ideal body weight in ounces of room temperature water for 2 weeks.
- Drink 8–12 ounces of water 15–30 minutes before each meal.

Eat More Seasonal and Alkaline Foods

- Look at the seasonal grocery lists in Appendix A and circle the foods for each season that you love. Give yourself permission to eat more of those foods.
- When trying to decongest the lymph, emphasize the alkaline foods and reduce the foods from the acidic foods list.
- Emphasize berries, beets, and colorful roots like turmeric, leafy greens, and seeds like fennel, chia and flax. Citrus fruits, including their pith, make great lymph-moving foods.

Lymph-Moving Herbs

- Consider supplementing with herbs like manjistha, nettles, dandelion, turmeric, ocotillo, queen's root, astragalus, red root, brahmi (also known as *Centella asiatica* or gotu kola), and fennel and nettles as teas.

Lymph-Moving Exercise
- All exercise is good for the lymph. Rebounding and safely-performed inverted yoga postures are particularly beneficial for the lymph.
- See Chapter 13 for your lymph-moving, digestion-rebooting *Eat Wheat* Workout.

Avoid Wheat and Dairy Until Lymph is Moving
- Cleansing the lymph is Step 1 towards being able to digest wheat and dairy again. Step 2 is to reboot the upper digestion, which is the topic of Chapter 10.

Looking Ahead
Now that we have discussed how to support our lymphatic systems for optimal health and digestive function, let's explore in Chapter 10 how to turn on the upper digestive system and start digesting wheat and dairy once again!

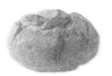

Chapter 10
FINDING YOUR
CAST IRON STOMACH

A patient in the U.K. recently wrote me an email in hopes that I share her letter in this book.

Dear Dr. John,

About 5 years ago, I started to suffer from incredible swelling of the stomach, combined with all sorts of digestive problems ranging from stomach gurgling to occasional constipation, diarrhea, and mucus in the stool, which I just lived with and got on with.

Then things started to get progressively worse. I went to the doctor and they asked me to make a food diary to help identify what foods were causing my problems. To start with, I thought it was wheat/gluten, so I tried eliminating this from my diet, but found that I was still having problems. At that point, I thought it could be a dairy intolerance. My doctor's advice was to eliminate the foods causing the problem from my diet and gradually reintroduce them.

My other symptoms at the time were that my immune system must have been seriously compromised, as during this time I had shingles (I'm not sure if it has the same name in the U.S., but it's also known as herpes zoster) and many colds/chest infections. I also experienced an episode where I woke up in the middle of the night struggling to breathe and the doctors diagnosed me with mild asthma. In addition, I had mucus in my stools, but didn't REALIZE that this was not normal!

Eliminating certain foods from my diet didn't really have any effect on my symptoms, and it got to the point where, after 1 night out with friends in summer 2014, I had eaten pasta carbonara and, once home, became violently sick with diarrhea.

At this point I knew something had to be done. I was assessed by a doctor and had a range of blood tests performed. I was told that everything was fine. I am generally a healthy, slim person. Of the 20+ different blood tests performed, only one came back outside of the normal levels, but I was told that this one was clinically insignificant. It was my bilirubin levels.

Given this was the professional advice; I thought nothing more of it. Coincidentally, that weekend I read an article in the Sunday Times talking about digestive disorders and how people could benefit from taking digestive enzymes. On the surface, this seemed to be the answer to my problems, but the more I thought about it, the more counterintuitive it seemed to have to take something as a supplement that your body should be producing itself.

I therefore Googled "should I be taking digestive enzymes?" and one of the first articles that came up was one written by you, stating that no, you shouldn't, and giving the reasons why. I then looked into what bilirubin levels are all about—its relationship to bile and the digestive process, and the whole picture fell into place, thanks to your article.

I read up on all the articles in your LifeSpa website and ordered triphala and manjistha, which I have taken since.

As you may have guessed, my body type is vata and my food intake was variable as I was often too busy to eat and when I did, I wasn't eating properly. I now ensure that I take the time for meals and eat as well as I can. I am now able to tolerate any food and all my digestive problems seem to have gone.

There is 1 final part to this story, and I am only telling you this to complete the picture, as it may have a bearing on all of the above. Last month, I was diagnosed with breast cancer and I am now undergoing a course of chemo. I have been told that my chances of survival are excellent and my treatment (chemo, surgery, and radiotherapy) should cure the cancer.

I want to finish by telling you how grateful I am to you, as without your article I would still be experiencing the digestive problems and many other health issues. I am now trying to follow the Ayurvedic diet as much as possible and I can hopefully go on to lead a long healthy life (I am 49).

With kind regards and many thanks,
Connie[6]

When your digestion begins to unravel and you are experiencing signs of indigestion and discomfort, it is important to remove hard-to-digest foods from you diet, just as Connie did. Generally, this will offer some relief, as we are making life a bit easier for the digestive process. Once the digestive problem is solved, these foods can be slowly reintroduced back into the diet. However, they should be non-processed, prepared properly, organic, and in season.

At the end of Connie's letter, she mentioned how she skips meals and eats on the run. Once again, I cannot emphasize enough the importance of eating in a relaxed manner. Be sure to take time, sit down, relax, and enjoy your meal. Connie was stressed, and the stress irritated her gut to the point where she was producing so much intestinal mucus that she could see it in her stool.

Connie had many signs of lymphatic congestion, ranging from her herpes (shingles) to her compromised immune system in the form of colds, chest infections, and her breathing difficulty. We discussed these and other symptoms of lymphatic congestion in Chapter 4.

As a result of years with a congested lymphatic system, the liver itself can become congested, and bile flow and production can be compromised. The

6　All names of patients have been changed throughout this book to protect their privacy, and all patients have given permission to share the story of their health journey in this book.

stomach—whose job it is to produce acid to break down things like wheat and dairy—depends on adequate bile to buffer the acid that the stomach produces. In Connie's case, her stomach decided to hold onto the food as long as possible in an attempt to wait for the bile to be released by the gallbladder. While she had battled with intestinal inflammation and lymphatic congestion for years, it was the logjam in her liver, gallbladder and/or bile ducts that triggered most of her problems.

The sad part of the story for Connie was that, after all she had been through, she was diagnosed with breast cancer. Breast cancer is almost always related to some type of lymphatic congestion. This is a perfect example of why I am so adamant about rebooting the digestive strength we were meant to have throughout our lives. Poor digestion equals poor detoxification, and when the lymph system becomes overwhelmed with toxins, the body becomes much more vulnerable to more serious health concerns.

Digestion and Detoxification

Our first line of defense against a toxic environment and our ability to convert hard-to-digest foods into nutrients requires a very robust upper digestive system. This requires a coordinated effort between the nervous system, which must be relaxed and calm to sense, with the five senses, what type of food is about to be eaten.

Digestive enzymes are released upon the first sight and smell of food. This is followed by a coordinated digestive response from the stomach's production of acid and pepsin, adequate production of bile from the liver, and the ability to deliver that bile into the small intestine. The production and delivery of pancreatic enzymes, the coordination of duodenal enzymes, and of course, the creation of an environment based on all the above that supports a healthy upper digestive microbiome are directly responsible for the complete breakdown of hard-to-digest foods like wheat and dairy.

Our Modern Digestion

In Connie's case, her liver was clearly congested and her bile was either not being produced in sufficient quantities or it had become too thick, sluggish, and viscous. Thick, viscous, and congested bile does not often show up on an ultrasound scan of the gallbladder.

Since the gallbladder's bile duct and the pancreatic duct that transports enzymes physically join together before entering the small intestine, congested bile can cause both poor digestive enzyme and bile flow.

As a result, just taking digestive enzymes may make the digestive symptoms better, but Connie wanted to finally get to the root of her health issues and heal from the inside out, not just treat her symptoms. Rarely is the problem a need for digestive enzyme supplementation due to an irreversible lack of pancreatic enzyme production, as is commonly touted. Congestion and inflammation of the bile and pancreatic ducts is typically the culprit. Without optimal flow of bile and pancreatic enzymes, neither digestion nor detoxification function optimally.

In addition, both bile and pancreatic enzymes are major buffers for the HCl in the stomach. If there are no buffers in the small intestine, the stomach will simply hold onto the acid, causing the stomach to swell or cause heartburn and a host of other signs of indigestion. The stomach can also literally decrease the production of the acid. Without the production of a very strong concentration of HCl in the stomach, proteins like casein, soy, wheat, and others will simply not be initially broken down in the upper digestion completely.

Does your Bile Need a Reboot?

If you answer "yes" to 1 or more of the questions below, your liver or gallbladder may need support:

1.	Do you ever get nauseous after a meal?	Yes or No
2.	Do you ever feel heavy after a high-fat meal?	Yes or No
3.	Do you ever get occasional heartburn after a meal?	Yes or No
4.	Do you have trouble digesting wheat, dairy, soy corn or nuts?	Yes or No
5.	Do you ever have sluggish, green, or greasy stools?	Yes or No
6.	Do you have a history of any gallbladder problems?	Yes or No

The gallbladder is a vital organ that stores concentrated bile to be able to help digest good fats, process bad fats and toxins, maintain healthy bowel movements, and buffer the digestive acids from the stomach.[493, 494] As I mentioned, if the liver becomes congested as a result of toxins, stress, and/or poor diet and elimination, the bile in the gallbladder can become thick, viscous and congested. In an attempt to keep the thick bile flowing, MRI findings commonly show that bile ducts dilate beyond what is considered normal while liver function is maintained within normal ranges.[495] Thick bile affects the ability to digest and detoxify, to maintain healthy weight and mood, and our overall health and vitality.[494, 496-498]

In Chapter 9, I discussed how beets, green vegetables and apples help support healthy lymph function. I'd like to devote the rest of this chapter to these and other rockstar foods and herbs that also support the liver and gallbladder (and therefore healthy bile production). You'll find these foods and spices also come with some additional amazing side benefits!

You Can't Beat Beets

Beets are my favorite go-to food to boost liver function and lymph and bile flow, and they also have some unexpected benefits that are making news. Red beet juice has become the preferred performance-enhancing drink for the Auburn College football team, and based on a handful of compelling studies, beet juice has even made it to the NFL, recommended by the Houston Texans as their pre-game drink![499]

Beets happen to be one of the highest sources of performance-enhancing nitrates. Yes, nitrates from plants such as beets, celery, and cauliflower are actually good for you, while nitrates found in packaged meats such as bacon, sausage, hot dogs, deli meats, packaged ham, pepperoni, and salami are quite toxic.

Plant-based nitrates in the diet convert easily into nitrites, which have a powerful vasodilation effect; helpful for opening up congested bile ducts. Vasodilation also refers to the widening of blood and lymphatic vessels, resulting in better circulation and lymph drainage of toxins, more efficient delivery of oxygen and nutrients to the cells, as well as improved physical performance.[500] Poor blood flow due to a lack of healthy vasodilation may be a factor in the decline of physical and cognitive function associated with aging.[500]

Many studies are currently underway reviewing the potential health benefits of nitrites and beet supplements.[500] One study demonstrated that running performance was significantly improved by supplementing with beet juice.[501] All of these findings suggest that beets are not only great for upper digestive bile flow but support circulation, oxygenation and lymphatic drainage for every cell in the body.[499-501]

Beet juice also increases cerebral circulation to certain parts of the brain that govern executive function, suggesting that beets may also support the drainage of the newly discovered lymph that drain toxins from the brain.[5, 500] Executive function is what allows us to do things like organizing, planning, remembering details and managing time. As a vasodilator, the nitrates in beets may support healthy cognitive function and memory by enhancing blood supply and possible lymph drainage to and from specific areas of the brain.[500]

The vasodilation effects of beetroot have also been shown to support healthy blood pressure. In one study, drinking just 500ml of beet juice lowered blood pressure by 10 points in 3 hours, possibly due to the blood vessel-dilating and lymph-supporting effects of the nitrates in beets.[502]

Beets for a Liver and Bile Boost

Beets are also very rich in B vitamins, calcium, iron, and powerful antioxidants such as alpha-lipoic acid (ALA). All of these support healthy liver function and lymph and bile flow. Poor bile flow is extremely common and is linked to weak stomach acid, inadequate liver detoxification and poor fat metabolism,[203] all of which are required to digest wheat and dairy.

In one study, both beets and okra were found to attach to bile in the intestines.[503] Once the bile is attached to certain types of fiber, like beet fiber, its job is to escort the toxic bile to the toilet. This is important because bile, when attached to fiber, carries toxic cholesterol particles, environmental pollutants, and a variety of other fat-soluble toxins it picks up on its journey through the liver and intestines. Without adequate fiber, up to 94 percent of this toxic bile can be reabsorbed back to the liver and back into circulation.[203]

This is one of the reasons why I recommend blending over juicing. The cellulose fiber is mixed with the juice in blending, but removed in juicing. While there are benefits with juicing, it can supply the body with too much sugar and too little of the much-needed fiber.

Beets also provide powerful liver-protective support. In another study, mice that were fed beets for 10 days produced a large amount of the body's 2 most powerful antioxidant liver enzymes, superoxide dismutase and glutathione, which rid the body of toxins.[504] Both of these antioxidants have been found to be active in the lymphatic system and are found to reduce inflammation,[5, 9] which is the real culprit of most of the symptoms related to food intolerances and the "grain brain."[3]

Beets for a Blood Sugar-Balancing Boost

Surprisingly, beets—which are loaded with beet sugar—have been shown to help support healthy blood sugar levels in type 2 diabetics.[505] Much of these benefits can be attributed to the high levels of alpha-lipoic acid (ALA) found in beets, which seem to offset the effects of the beet sugar. ALA is both water- and fat-soluble, which allows it to penetrate any tissue in the body. For this reason, it has become a popular skincare ingredient. As an antioxidant, the ALA can support lymphatic movement in the body and help resolve free radical damage.[505] I'll discuss more about sugar in Chapter 11.

 Tip: When trying to boost bile production in the liver and bile flow from the gallbladder, try to eat 1 red beet a day. Beets increase bile flow, which helps move the bowels, so do not be alarmed if your elimination improves or the stool turns reddish color.

⊰⊱⊱ Beet Tonic Recipe ⊰⊰⊱

Ingredients:
- 1 fresh beet, peeled and grated
- Juice of 1/2 lemon
- 1 tablespoon olive oil—make sure it's extra virgin, cold-pressed, organic, and stamped with a harvest and/or bottling date.

Directions:

1. Combine all ingredients.
2. Take 1 beet's worth of this combination daily for 2–4 weeks to reset bile flow.

Green is Good

Green vegetables are the #1 food for the liver; leafy greens are loaded with micronutrients and minerals that the liver needs to function optimally. In addition to making an effort to have half of every meal as vegetables, here is a classic green tonic recipe that feeds and supports liver and gallbladder function.

⫸⫸⫸ Green Tonic Recipe ⫷⫷⫷

Ingredients:

- 1 bunch parsley
- 3 medium zucchini
- 1/2 pound green beans
- 5 stalks celery

Directions:

1. Steam all ingredients for just 8–10 minutes, and then mix in a blender. You can drink as a soup, or once cooled, as a tonic/smoothie. You can add water to get the desired consistency, as well as a good squeeze of fresh lemon juice.
2. Drink 1–3 green tonics per day as a meal or with meals, as needed for gallbladder pain and/or to optimize gallbladder function.
3. *Options for more flavor:* Any green vegetable can be substituted for the veggies above. Try adding a steamed apple. Or you can try adding garlic and ginger with low-sodium vegetable broth. Avocados add a nice creamy texture as well.

An Apple a Day

Consume at least 1 apple a day after meals to increase bile flow. Apples have high amounts of malic acid, which helps to open up and dilate the bile ducts. The more sour the apple, the more bile-moving malic acid exists.[506]

Malic acid, which is found in high concentrations in apples, cranberries, and tart cherries, has been shown to increase alkalinity systemically, which naturally increases lymphatic flow and detox capacity.[507] Malic acid supplementation has also been shown to break up calcium oxalate kidney stones, and many experts believe it breaks up gallstones as well.[508] Malic acid is also used in liver flushes to dilate the bile ducts. Dietary use of these fruits can be used to support optimal bile flow.

Like most foods, apples have been hybridized for thousands of years to be sweeter. So instead of choosing the sweetest apples, try to get the more tart apples that carry less sugar and more bile-moving malic acid.

Fenugreek Tea

Today, fenugreek may be a lesser-known spice, but it was once very common and highly revered. In one study, fenugreek was found to reduce gallstones by 75 percent when participants were fed a high cholesterol diet for 10 weeks.[509] Fat levels in the liver as well as cholesterol levels also decreased with fenugreek. Researchers also found that fenugreek increased bile acid content in the bile, making for much more potent bile and lowered liver enzymes,[509] which suggest that the liver processed the high cholesterol diet with ease. The overall result of adding fenugreek to your diet is much healthier and thinner bile. Fenugreek is also well-studied to lower blood sugar. This tea with meals may help prevent the sugar belly I discuss in Chapter 11. You can buy the seeds and make a tea to drink with each meal to increase bile function and liver support, or grind or buy it as a spice to cook with. You can mix it with fennel seeds for the lymph and intestinal skin and make fennel, fenugreek tea.

⫸⫸ **Fenugreek Tea Recipe** ⫷⫷

Ingredients:
- 1 teaspoon fenugreek seeds
- 1 cup water
- Milk (optional)
- Nutmeg (optional)
- Lemon (optional)

Directions:
1. Use 1 teaspoon of fenugreek seeds for each cup of tea. Lightly crush fenugreek seeds with a large wooden spoon or the side of a chef's knife to release flavor and health benefits.
2. Place crushed fenugreek seeds into a tea strainer. (Add 1 teaspoon of whole fennel seeds to make fenugreek-fennel tea.)
3. Place the tea strainer into a small pan and add approximately 1 cup of water per teaspoon of seeds. Simmer for 2–3 minutes and steep for an additional 10–15 minutes. (Fenugreek seeds take longer to brew into tea than many other herbs or spices.)
4. Serve the tea hot or cold, adding sweetener or milk to taste. You may need to reheat before serving hot. Try enhancing with freshly grated nutmeg and a twist of lemon.

Bile Duct Cleanse

Shilajit is one of Ayurveda's most prized herbal medicines. It is the only herb in the *Materia Medica of Ayurveda*[510] that is labeled a panacea, indicating that it has a beneficial role to play in the health of all the systems of the body. Perhaps one of its most important properties is its ability to break up scar tissue and stones as a result of its high fulvic acid concentration. It is also known for delivering micronutrients into the deep tissues of the body for energy and longevity.[511] Traditionally, it was used to optimize liver function and the movement of bile from the liver and gallbladder. I use it effectively to help chelate toxins out of the body as well as to cleanse both the pancreatic and bile ducts for a deep, health-promoting cleaning.[512]

The Wonder of Turmeric

For liver and gallbladder function, lymph support, and repair and maintenance of the intestinal skin, turmeric may be the most researched herbal spice. As a natural anti-inflammatory and antioxidant for the liver, it has been shown in many studies to boost bile flow and bile production, but its magic extends well beyond the liver.[513]

 Reminder: Turmeric is high in oxalates, which can combine with calcium and form calcium oxalate stones in the kidney or gallbladder. Folks at risk for calcium oxalate kidney or gallstones should avoid turmeric and use my other suggestions to boost your bile flow.

Turmeric is also one of the most researched herbs for intestinal permeability or leaky gut syndrome. It has been shown to support the healthy function of the intestinal skin and healthy microbiome, which in turn supports both better intestinal integrity and digestive power.[232, 514]

One of the problems with turmeric is that it is difficult for the body to absorb. That is why many of the studies have been done on curcumin, which is the extract of turmeric and easier to absorb.

While modern herbal extracts have potent therapeutic value, it is difficult to match the blueprint of the original plant found in whole herbs and spices. Additionally, the process of extraction uses alcohol, which kills the beneficial microbes that actually live on whole organic plants. Whole herbs and spices carry specific microbes that support the actions of that plant, meaning the ingestion of the whole plant is necessary to deliver all of the plant's benefits. In addition, the body may build a tolerance to an extract. Whole herbs and spices, while not as potent as extracts, are foods and have a sustainable effect. In Ayurveda, whole herbs and spices are combined with other whole herbs and spices to boost function, which can be as potent as today's modern extracts.

Cooking with turmeric has been traditional in many parts of the world for thousands of years. When you combine 16 parts turmeric to 1 part black pepper, this combination can boost the assimilation of turmeric by a whopping 2,000 percent.[515] Curry is formulated in a similar ratio. This research was one of the first sources showing how turmeric could have so many medicinal powers once it had some help (from black pepper) being absorbed through the intestinal wall into the bloodstream and lymph.

What is interesting is that in India, curry powder is loaded with turmeric, peppers, and other spices. Turmeric is added to many dishes in India, and during the cooking process, the turmeric is naturally extracted and concentrated. In fact, the average person in India eats about 2–2.5 grams of turmeric a day—that's equivalent to about 4–6 capsules of turmeric a day—almost every day of their lives. Interestingly, India has among the lowest rates of prostate, breast, colon and lung cancer. Some researchers believe this may be due to the quantity of turmeric consumed on a regular basis.

Turmeric for the Brain

Perhaps one of our biggest concerns as we age is to find ways to protect ourselves from the ravages of cognitive decline. Turmeric has at least 10 neuro-protective actions that support healthy cognitive function.[516]

Because the brain is predominately fatty tissue, fat-soluble toxins may accumulate in the brain and cause damage. As a fat-soluble substance, turmeric may have an affinity for chelating (removing) fat-soluble toxins out of the deep tissues. Turmeric crosses the blood-brain barrier, where it may attach to neurotoxins, such as beta-amyloid plaque, and support healthy antioxidant activity.[517]

New studies, as described in Chapter 4, have found lymph vessels in the brain that drain toxins like beta-amyloid plaque, linked to Alzheimer's disease.[5] Turmeric has been shown to support healthy lymphatic flow, which may be the mechanism of how this herb has such tremendous benefit in supporting brain function and the brain fog associated with gluten sensitivity.[5, 468]

Turmeric for Mood Stability

New studies on turmeric have been exploring its effect on healthy and stable mood. In one study, curcumin was shown to boost the brain chemical norepinephrine, which supports healthy mood, attentiveness, sleep, dreaming, and higher learning.[518]

Perhaps surprisingly, curcumin also boosted levels of dopamine—the "motivation" hormone that supports pleasure, emotion, satisfaction and locomotion—and serotonin, which plays a key role in mood, memory, learning, appetite, sexual behavior, sleep, and many other functions.[518]

Turmeric is also believed to act as a brain-derived neurotrophic factor, which means it supports the growth and development of neurons and resists the degeneration of brain cells when under stress.[518]

Bile-Boosting Foods

In addition to supporting the body, brain, and bile with herbs and spices, there are many foods that help the liver produce more bile while maintaining the integrity of good healthy bile delivery into the small intestine.

Bile-Moving and Cholagogue Foods		
The following are foods that offer natural support for the function of the liver, gallbladder, and bile flow. To support your health, increase your consumption of these bile-moving or cholagogue foods:		
• Garlic	• Apples	• Olive oil
• Beets	• Avocado	• Ginger
• Celery	• Chicory	• Mustard Greens
• Ginger	• Black radish	• Turnip greens
• Coconut oil	• Dandelion	• Peppermint
• Artichoke	• Berries	• Leafy greens
• Hibiscus	• Lemon	• Cranberries

It's Time to turn on the Digestive Furnace

When folks complain about gas, bloating, or food intolerances, many experts often suggest HCl (hydrochloric acid) supplements. It is true that the HCl that is manufactured in the stomach can be depleted and cause a host of digestive issues. All proteins and especially gluten, dairy, and the anti-nutrients that surround and protect beans, soy, and nuts require a very strong stomach acid, or HCl, to be initially broken down and digested. So when these symptoms are present, giving HCl seems to make sense.

The body, however, is not equipped with gas gauges that measure HCl, digestive enzymes, or hormones for that matter, so it's tricky sometimes to know when our levels are low or when we may need a refill. There is always a reason why the body becomes depleted or stops producing enough HCl. If we just take HCl supplements and the body had a good reason why it stopped producing it, we can actually make things worse. The body is very intelligent and does what it does for a reason.

One of the most common reasons why the stomach would stop producing HCl is because the buffers—which include bile from the liver and gallbladder as well as digestive enzymes from the pancreas and small intestine—are not sufficient to buffer the acids needed to digest hard-to-digest proteins. The stomach can respond to this by dialing down the acid production. So before you add more HCl through supplementation, you need to make sure the bile is flowing.

This is why we troubleshoot the liver and gallbladder first. Once bile flow has been restored, you can then successfully turn on the stomach acid. I prefer herbs and spices over HCl supplementation to reboot the body's HCl production, as herbs train the body to do the job and avoid the risk of the body becoming dependent on digestive supplements.

"On- the-go" techniques to turn up the stomach's HCl production

- **Tip 1:** Drink 8–12 ounces of room temperature water 15–30 minutes before each meal.
- **Tip 2:** Add a pinch of salt and/or a pinch of black pepper to a large glass of water, and drink it 15–30 minutes before the meal. Both of these condiments boost digestive fire naturally. Conveniently, every restaurant has salt and pepper right on the table.
- **Tip 3:** Get fancy and order a cup of hot water with lemon first thing when eating out, or add a squeeze of lemon to the pre-meal water.

Typically, you may wait 15 minutes before the food arrives, which allows the water to prehydrate the stomach lining that buffers stomach acid, and the lemon juice helps to increase HCl production.

- **Tip 4:** Order a salad with the classic dressing of oil and vinegar. The oil increases bile flow from the liver and gallbladder, and the vinegar is acidic, which increases HCl acid production naturally.

- **Tip 5:** Sip hot water during the meal. This helps keep the food you are eating in a soupy consistency, which allows the HCl to more easily break down all the food in the stomach. Too much water during the meal can dilute your stomach acid, so don't overdrink. Avoid cold, iced drinks.

5 Digestive Spices to the Rescue

In addition to the above HCl-boosting techniques, I also suggest some ongoing upper digestive support to help permanently reset function. Whole, organic spices have been used for thousands of years for cooking, and delivering time-tested health benefits that are now well supported by science.

For example, there is compelling research and thousands of years of clinical use to suggest 5 digestive spices—fennel, coriander, cumin, cardamom, and ginger—deliver significant benefits for gas, bloating, and rebooting the natural strength of the digestive system,[519-525] as you will see below. Perhaps the most profound aspect of these spices is how gentle yet powerful they are. I find that even folks with the most sensitive digestive systems can do well on these 5 spices.

Chewing a handful of cumin, fennel, cardamom, and coriander seeds after a meal is still a common practice in India. This is why you will often find a bowl of fennel seeds awaiting you at the door as you exit your favorite Indian restaurant.

For re-training the body to digest wheat and dairy again, I find these 5 spices invaluable. Numerous studies suggest that cumin, fennel, cardamom, coriander and ginger build digestive self-sufficiency in these ways:

- Increase bile flow (no need for bile salts)[519]
- Increase pancreatic enzyme activity (no need for digestive enzymes)[519]
- Increase small intestine enzyme activity (no need for digestive enzyme supplements)[519]

- Decrease gas and bloating (no need for HCl supplements)[520]
- Increase fat and sugar metabolism[519]
- Are powerful free radial scavengers[521]
- Support optimal weight[522]
- Support microbiology health (especially ginger)[520]
- Improve gut health[520]
- Support a healthy growth rate of good bacteria (especially ginger)[520]
- Discourage H. pylori from adhering to stomach[522]
- Are digestive stimulants[523]
- Quicken the transit time in the intestines, supporting better elimination[521]

What is fascinating about these studies is that these 5 spices seem to support the body's natural ability to digest, rather than just treat its problematic symptoms. For example, while the studies show that these spices improved fat and sugar metabolism, they seem to do so by boosting more bile acid and pancreatic enzyme flow.[519, 523, 524]

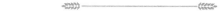

Digestive enzyme supplements provide the enzymes we need to digest protein and starches, while these spices amp up the body's *own* production of digestive enzymes and bile.[519, 523] This is an example of resetting digestion, rather than brewing dependency on digestive aids.

To further illustrate this point, in one study, ginger was shown to support healthier cells of the intestinal wall as well as boost the proliferation of good microbes in the gut, many of which are responsible for digesting gluten.[520] In another study, these spices blocked the bacterium H. pylori—linked to indigestion and stomach ulcers—from proliferating and adhering to the stomach lining.[522] The spices seem to work with the body's digestive intelligence by supporting better digestive function, a healthier environment for the digestive microbes, healthier villi and improved intestinal function.[519-521]

Cooking with these spices is a great way to make the meal more digestible, or you can take these spices in capsule form before meals to boost digestion. Alternatively, they can be made into a tea to have with the meal.

The 5 Spices of Digestion: Up Close and Personal

The magic of these spices takes place when they are all taken together to boost digestive strength. They each have well-documented benefits as individual herbs or spices, but when they are combined, the result is quite another story. Let's take a look at these spices individually.

Coriander Seed (Coriandrum sativum)

- Coriander is perhaps the most cooling of the 5 digestive spices. The seeds are commonly used in herbal medicine for a host of ailments; the leaves are commonly known as cilantro. The seeds are best known for their digestive properties by cooling excess heat, inflammation or digestive acid in the body and intestinal tract, and are thus soothing for the digestive tract. Therefore, coriander is used effectively for occasional heartburn. It is a natural carminative, which means it prevents or relieves gas from the intestinal tract, and is beneficial for numerous heat-related conditions in the body.[526]

Cardamom (Elettaria cardamomum)

- As a member of the ginger family, Ayurvedic texts celebrated cardamom's ability to make foods easier to digest and enhance the taste of most ordinary foods.[525]
- Its taste is most recognizable in a cup of Indian chai tea, allowing the chai to boost the digestive process. Cardamom is known to reduce the extreme acidity of many foods and caffeinated beverages, including coffee; it is also the signature spice in traditional Turkish coffee. When cooked into your food, it reduces excess mucus, gas and bloating in the stomach and small intestine while supporting healthy blood sugar and cholesterol levels.[525]

Cumin Seed (**Cuminum cyminum**)

- Cumin is perhaps the most powerful digestive tonic of the 5 spices of digestion. It has a strong taste and, while very effective alone, it blends well in both taste and effectiveness with the other 4 spices for boosting digestion and reducing gas and bloating. It is much like coriander in that it cools the digestive system while boosting digestive strength. It supports healthy assimilation and the proliferation of good microbes, as well as the detoxification of the intestinal tract.[527]

Fennel Seed (**Foeniculum vulgare**)

Fennel not only combats gas and bloating in the digestive tract, it is one of Ayurveda's favorite lymph-movers. As a lymph-mover, it supports new mothers' healthy lactation and radiant skin on both the outside and inside (intestinal skin). It has a strong balancing effect on all types of bodies and constitutions. It is one of the best herbs for digestion, as it strengthens the digestive fire without aggravating excess heat, and is beneficial for intestinal cramping, nausea, and dispelling flatulence.[528]

Ginger Root (**Zingiber officinale**)

In Ayurveda, ginger is called "the universal spice" because of its many health benefits. It is heating for the upper digestion with its pungent taste, but cooling and soothing for the lower digestion as a result of its sweet aftertaste. It is the classic kindling to start the digestive fire in the stomach. Scientific studies have shown that it supports healthy microbes, a healthy intestinal wall, and acts as a digestive stimulant for nutrient assimilation.[520]

Tip: For best results, do one of the following:
- Mix these 5 spices and encapsulate them.
- Sprinkle 1/2 teaspoon on your food.
- Cook with this mixture or make a tea out of them to drink with the meal.
- You can make a tea in the same way you did with the fenugreek seeds previously mentioned.

- You can also find this combination in a capsule form at LifeSpa. com called Gentle Digest.

Resetting Digestive Fire

Once the bile is flowing optimally and the digestion and elimination have been strengthened, it is sometimes necessary to relight the stomach's digestive acid production. The following technique is for stubborn, boggy digestion with chronic gas and bloating and no heartburn symptoms at all. *Again, this technique is for wet, boggy and dull upper digestion—not overly hot or acidic digestion.*

The classical Ayurvedic formula used for this procedure, called trikatu, is made up of equal parts pippali (long pepper), ginger, and black pepper. These spices work synergistically to stimulate the digestive fire, allowing for more efficient digestion in the stomach while promoting proper bile flow, healthy detoxification and fat metabolism. The gentle heating action of this blend primes the digestive tract to digest food, absorb nutrients, and efficiently remove wastes.[529-535]

 Reminder: If there is a tendency for heartburn, or the digestion is sensitive, do not use trikatu—use the "5-spice mixture," described earlier.

Digestive Fire Reset Protocol

You are going to take increasing amounts of capsules of trikatu (or the 5-spice mixture) before each meal until you feel a comfortable warmth around your belly. Then, you will slowly decrease each dose by 1 capsule while maintaining the sensation of warmth.

 Tip: You can find the formula, Trikatu in most health food stores or as Warm Digest at LifeSpa.com along with the 5 spices formula in capsules, as Gentle Digest.

- Take 1 capsule before breakfast.
- Take 2 capsules before lunch.

- Take 3 capsules before supper.
- Take 4 the next day before breakfast.

Continue until you find your *Maximum Dose* (details below). Do not take more than 6 capsules at a time.

Note: If there is any pain or discomfort at any time during this reset, stop the protocol and read the upcoming section on heartburn.

Finding Your Maximum Dose

Keep adding 1 capsule before each meal until you begin to feel some warmth around your belly—either before, during, or after the meal. This is your Maximum Dose. You may feel warmth after taking 2 capsules or after taking 6. Do not take more than 6 capsules.

If you experience any burning or loose stools at any time and no warmth around your belly, consider this the limit and stop increasing the digestive herbs.

Start Decreasing While Maintaining the Warmth

Once you feel the warmth in or around your belly, begin to decrease your dose by 1 capsule at the next meal. Continue taking this until you feel heat again. This may take 1–2 meals, or even a few days.

Once you feel warmth again, decrease by 1 capsule at the next meal and continue this dose until you feel warmth again. Continue this protocol until you have weaned down to 1 capsule and then to no capsules at all. You may need to stay at 1 capsule for a few weeks.

Example Patient

She began to feel warmth in and around her belly on the second day after breakfast while taking 4 capsules of trikatu. This was her maximum dose. At her next meal (lunch), she decreased to 3 capsules and took this dose until she felt warmth again the next day (also at lunch). She then decreased to 2 capsules before each meal until she felt warmth again the following day at breakfast. At breakfast, she decreased to 1 capsule and continued that dose for 3 days until she felt warmth.

How it Works

This protocol is designed to reset your digestive furnace, which is often too weak due to stress or other digestive imbalances. The warmth felt around the belly is a sign that the digestive spices are helping the stomach increase production of HCl (hydrochloric acid). Slowly decreasing the dose of the spices based on when you feel warmth ensures that your stomach continues to produce HCl and your digestive fire stays abundant even when you wean down to 1 capsule before meals and, finally, completely stop taking the herbs.

Heartburn: A Sign of Weak Digestion

For the body to break down gluten, it must have a strong, balanced stomach acid (HCl) production. The stomach acid is the trigger for the rest of the digestive process. If the HCl is too high or low, then the ability to digest gluten will be compromised. Let's make sure the stomach acid is optimal before we begin to reintroduce foods like wheat and dairy back into the diet. Please see your MD if your heartburn symptoms persist.

There are many types of heartburn, but commonly, the acid-burning feeling is part of a condition known as GERD (Gastroesophageal Reflux Disease). This is caused by stomach acid building up in the stomach and refluxing or moving up into the esophagus, irritating the esophageal lining. This can cause burning, an acid taste in the mouth, coughing, wheezing, hoarseness, ulcers, cancer and/or pain.

GERD is a chronic problem. When it happens over time, the lower esophageal sphincter (LES), which separates the stomach from the esophagus, fails to function optimally, and acid is allowed to reflux up into and irritate the delicate tissue lining the esophagus.

The conventional understanding is that excess production of stomach acid (HCl) causes heartburn. When HCl is produced in excess, it will burn the stomach lining and, in the case of GERD, the esophageal lining as well.

Excess spicy foods as well as citric fruits, tomatoes, garlic, onions, hot spices, sugar, rich foods, and fried foods can all contribute to the excess production of stomach acid and heartburn. Chronic stress will trigger the release of excess cortisol, a stress hormone, which stimulates the release of excess stomach acid as well and can also cause heartburn.

The Low HCl Heartburn

While excess HCl is a major cause of heartburn, heartburn symptoms may not be caused by too much acid, but too little! That's right; heartburn can be caused by not *enough* acid production in the stomach. If there is too little stomach acid produced, the food and the stomach acid (even though there is less of it) will linger in the stomach and delay the emptying. The longer the food sits in the stomach, the higher the risk of irritation to the stomach lining.

Imagine all the foods you eat entering into a stomach that had little or no acid to break it down. In short order, the foods would be an irritant to the stomach lining. In a low-acid stomach environment, undesirable microbes such as H. pylori that are often synonymous with heartburn can proliferate and irritate and further inflame the stomach lining, causing low acid-related heartburn.[536]

Common Causes of Too Little Acid

- Reduction of stomach acid due to lack of bile flow.
- Eating excess over-processed foods that are difficult to digest, depleting stomach acid.
- Eating while stressed will initially increase cortisol and increase stomach acid. But over time, with chronic stress, the cortisol will underperform and acid production will be less than adequate.
- Drinking large amounts of cold beverages or alcohol with meals.
- Overeating at night will bog down the digestive fire.
- Eating excess heavy and rich foods will bog down the digestive fire.

Determine Your Type of Heartburn Quiz

- ***Too Much Acid:*** Mix 1/4 teaspoon of baking soda in 1 cup (8 ounces) of water and drink during acid symptoms. If the burning is caused by too much acid, the baking soda—which is extremely alkaline—will buffer the acids and relieve the pain.
- ***Too Little Acid:*** Mix 1 tablespoon of apple cider vinegar in 8 ounces of water and drink this during acid symptoms. This will increase acid and reduce the burning if this is due to too little acid.

Insufficient Bile Flow

If the heartburn is caused by insufficient bile flow from the liver or gallbladder, the heartburn usually kicks in at night, or 30–60 minutes after a meal. This happens because it takes some time for the stomach acid to build up and/or spill small amounts of acid into the small intestine that has produced inadequate amounts of bile to buffer it.

Eating heavy, rich, fatty or fried foods—more so than spicy foods—can cause heartburn due to a lack of bile flow. This is because bile is responsible for the breakdown of fats. If there is inadequate bile flow, the fatty meal will sit in the stomach undigested and burn, causing burping or nausea.

Can't Digest Anything? Check Your Pancreatic Enzymes

Pancreatic enzymes are involved in digesting fats, proteins and carbs so a lack of these enzymes can cause just about any type of indigestion. The best way to explore your own pancreatic enzyme balance is to take some over-the-counter digestive enzymes and, if you feel better after taking them, you can deduce that the bile ducts that carry the bile and pancreatic enzymes are likely congested. As we have discussed, the beets, apples, fenugreek, turmeric and 5-spice mixture are all excellent to open up those ducts.

Strategies to Address Heartburn with Low Acid

In Chapter 9, I discussed the use of apple cider vinegar (ACV) to be used in supporting the body in many ways, such as moving lymphatic congestion and boosting HCl production. Taking 1 tablespoon of ACV with 8 ounces of water 15–30 minutes before meals can be used for heartburn caused by either too little or too much stomach acid. ACV has been shown to reduce heartburn, increase digestive strength, balance blood sugar and mitigate many of the symptoms of gluten intolerance.[482, 483]

When heartburn is caused by low HCl production, it is commonly due to poor bile flow as well. Follow the food, herb and spice recommendations I described above to boost bile flow.

Strategies To Address Heartburn with High Acid[262]

When stomach acid is too high, I suggest the following strategies (discussed in detail in Chapters 8 and 9):

- **Apple Cider Vinegar**—Can be used for too low or high HCl production
- **5 Spices**—Can be used to balance HCl, bile and enzyme production
- **Amalaki**—Supports healthy repair of the intestinal skin
- **Brahmi (*Centella asiatica*)**—Cooling and helps repair stomach and intestinal lining
- **Colonizing probiotics**—Restores a healthy microbiology found to support digestion
- **Slippery Elm**—Protects stomach lining from acid irritation
- **Marshmallow Root**—Protects stomach lining from acid irritation
- **Licorice Root**—Protects stomach lining from acid irritation

Upper Digestive Complications: Stomach Pulling

In Ayurveda, there is a condition called "udvarta," where stomach acid builds up in the stomach and is forced up into the esophagus causing heartburn, GERD, or acid reflux. Over time, this condition can cause the stomach to press up onto the diaphragm instead of hanging freely from it. There are many reasons for this condition, including stress, poor elimination, poor bile flow, and excess stomach acid.

In some cases, the upward pressure of the stomach can cause irritation, inflammation, and pain on the abdomen just under the rib cage. In extreme cases, it can adhere itself to the underside of the diaphragm, rendering the stomach unable to digest hard-to-digest foods like wheat, dairy and fatty foods. With part of the stomach bound to the diaphragmatic wall, this can a make it harder for the stomach to effectively empty the stomach's contents into the small intestine.

In severe situations, the stomach can put so much pressure on the diaphragm that it can actually herniate through the diaphragm and cause a common condition called hiatal hernia. Where the esophagus passes through the diaphragm, there is a sphincter called the lower esophageal sphincter, which opens and closes, which allows food to pass through and keeps acid out. After years of upward pressure, this sphincter gives out and part of the stomach pushes up through the diaphragm.

Some of the symptoms associated with upward digestive pressure:

- Hay fever
- Occasional headaches
- Breakouts
- Brain fog
- Sore throats
- Occasional heartburn
- Indigestion
- Occasional constipation
- Weight gain
- Gluten intolerance
- Dairy intolerance
- Achy neck and shoulders
- Issues with the eyes, ears, nose and throat

Hanging out with the Stomach

The diaphragm is a big, flat muscle that separates your chest cavity from your abdomen and regulates breathing depth and patterns. The stomach is designed to hang underneath the diaphragm. But after years of:

- Stress
- Shallow breathing (through the mouth)
- Pregnancies (due to upward pressure from the baby pushing up on the stomach and diaphragm)
- Lack of exercise
- Lack of yoga, and
- Indigestion

...the diaphragm can begin to tighten and pull the stomach up towards itself. This is common after childbirth causing chronic post-partum digestive problems.

Getting Unstuck

To determine if you have this condition, take your thumb and press deeply under the left side of your rib cage and see if it is tender to touch. If it is painful, sore, tender, or hard in this area, you might have a stomach that is pressing unnaturally onto the diaphragm. You may also want to poke under the right side of the rib cage as well and see if that area is sore. The liver hangs closely next to the diaphragmatic surface on the right side; if it is sore, you may need to treat the right side as well.

Stomach Pulling Technique

1. Sit in a chair with a backrest, so your stomach muscles can relax. Take your left thumb and poke the abdomen just under the rib cage on your left side on the sore or tight area. Use your right thumb on top of your left to help put more pressure of the left thumb to push in more deeply. Soreness is an indication that you can benefit from this technique and that you are in the correct spot.

2. With your thumbs pressing into your stomach just under the rib cage, begin to lean forward. This will soften the tummy and allow you to push more deeply into the abdomen and stomach.

3. With your right and left thumbs, begin to pull downwards, towards your navel, in effect pulling your stomach downwards and separating it from the diaphragm.

4. As you are pulling downwards, take a big inhalation, continue pulling down on your stomach with your thumbs while you begin to lean back in your chair, arching your back. Be sure the abdominal muscles do not contract while you lean back. This will extend your back, leveraging the rib cage upwards as you pull the stomach downwards in the direction of the navel.

5. At the end of the inhale, lean forward again in your chair and exhale as you go all the way forward. Poke in again with the left thumb to find a sore or tight area; back it up with the right thumb and pull the stomach down. Inhale deeply again as you pull down with your thumbs and extend or arch your back.

6. Continue working your way across the left and right sides where you felt soreness or tension.

Continue this procedure for 2 minutes twice a day until the area is painless and supple. Be careful not to overdo it. Too much pressure can bruise the area and slow down the progress. The tenderness may take days or weeks to resolve.

 Tip: This may be easier to understand by watching a video. You can find an instructional video at http://lifespa.com/learn-stomach-pulling.

Additional Techniques to Release the Stomach-Diaphragm Tension and Optimize Digestive Function

Following are a few simple, yet effective tools that can help keep your stomach hanging in the proper way:

- **Nasal Breathing Exercise:** Deep nasal breathing during exercise is one of the best ways to expand the diaphragm and create space in the abdominal cavity. See Chapter 13 for instructions on Nasal Breathing Exercise.
- **Sun Salutations:** This series of yoga postures alternates extension and flexion, naturally stretching and massaging the region around the diaphragm and stomach junction. See Chapter 13 and Appendix D for instructions on Sun Salutations.
- **Hand Massage Vibrator:** Using a handheld electric massager, vibrate the area between the stomach and lower rib cage. Do this for 2 minutes twice a day until all the tenderness and tightness of both left and right sides of the sternum just below the rib cage are pain-free, soft, and supple. For best results, follow this with the stomach pulling technique.

The After-Meal Coma

Have you ever eaten a big meal and then used every ounce of energy you had not to fall asleep? Some of the lymphatic research I cited in Chapter 4 suggests that the lymphatic system can take a couple of hours to clear after digesting a meal. Weak digestion and a congested lymphatic system can slow the delivery of energy producing fats from the lymph to the muscles and brain and possibly cause after-meal fatigue or the famous "food coma."

During my Ayurvedic training in India, I remember eating a very large lunch with my teacher. We were at a conference and I knew if I went back into the hall I would fall asleep in my chair. I told my teacher I was going to lie down in my room and I would come back to the hall later. He quickly rebutted, telling me, "No, lay on your left side and I will come back in 10 minutes and we will go to the hall together and you will be fine."

I told him that I ate too much and I was sure to be asleep in 10 minutes, and if I did not answer the door to go to the hall without me. I went to my room and did as he told me. Strangely, when he came to my door I was awake, and we went to the hall together; even stranger, I was wide awake the entire afternoon listening to lectures in Hindi—which I cannot even understand!

After the meeting, I asked my teacher how that happened. I was so tired after such a big meal that I was nearly falling asleep at the table. He told me that we did overeat, but the food was fresh, prepared well, and we ate it in a relaxed way. He said what we ate, how we ate it and then resting on my left side after the meal helped me digest the food into energy. When people fall asleep after a meal, it is because of weak digestion. Once you fix the digestion, you can begin to enjoy larger, more relaxing mid-day meals without the food coma.

Relaxing while eating and then resting on the left side after a large meal is an age-old Ayurvedic technique to improve digestion that has been documented by modern science. For example, in one study, researchers measured alertness and task performance after groups took either no nap, a 15-minute nap, or a 45-minute nap after a large meal. The results agreed with the siesta principle: A short nap—as opposed to a long nap—is ideal. The group that took a 15-minute nap after the meal demonstrated better alertness 30 minutes—and up to 3 hours—after the meal. Task performance was also significantly better in the 15-minute nap group compared to the 45-minute and no-nap groups.[440]

Left Side, Best Side

The instruction to lie on your left side is also supported in a handful of other studies. When you lie on your left side after a meal, the stomach is cradled to allow the food to more effortlessly exit the stomach and enter the small intestine. When standing or lying on the right side, there is undue pressure on the pyloric sphincter, which may allow the food to exit the stomach prematurely, causing issues of indigestion, gas and bloating. In one study, babies fed while lying on their left side had better digestion and less colic, while other studies showed that lying on the left side helped ease occasional heartburn.[441, 442]

If you tend to get sleepy after a big meal, consider the following:

- Relax while eating the meal.
- Don't watch TV or be distracted while eating.
- Dine and enjoy light (not stressful) conversation.
- Rest on your left side for 10–15 minutes after the meal whenever possible.

- Take a stroll after the post-meal rest.
- Troubleshoot your lymph, gallbladder and stomach acid production.

Looking Ahead

Now that we have some tried-and-true tools for resetting and supporting our digestion, we have to address America's new pre-diabetic epidemic I call "Sugar Belly."

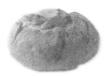

Chapter 11
SUGAR BELLY

I n my opinion, the idea of "wheat belly" would be better described as "sugar belly," since science has implicated sugar as the cause of the world's next great epidemic, "diabesity"—a combination of diabetes and obesity. Sugar is also the real culprit in the grain brain syndrome. David Perlmutter, M.D., the author of *Grain Brain,* describes Alzheimer's disease as type 3 diabetes where the high glycemic index of grains are link to poor brain health. As I mentioned in Chapter 1, the link to cognitive decline is sugar, and not necessarily wheat or grain.

Around the world, glutenous grains like wheat and barley have been staple foods for thousands[22]—even millions of years.[21, 64] When you peruse through history books, it is rare to see pictures of folks who were overweight. Even as recently as the 1950s and 1960s, when I grew up, overweight kids, attention deficit disorders, diabetes and gluten or dairy intolerances—all situations related to sugar consumption—were rarely seen compared to today.

In the 1960s, mass-produced and processed foods became the foundation of the new "Standard American Diet" (SAD), and with it came a host of health problems—pre-diabetes being one of them.[537, 538] Obesity, diabetes, ADD, asthma, depression, chronic fatigue, Alzheimer's disease and now non-celiac gluten sensitivity issues have reached all-time highs with no counter-trend in sight.

In general, processed foods are quicker to be broken down into sugar, or glucose, which enters the bloodstream much faster than whole foods. Excess sugar in the blood will trigger the release of excess insulin, which in turn converts and stores the excess sugar in the body in the form of unwanted fat and damaging cholesterol particles.

Perhaps more damaging is the effect of a degenerative process called glycation. This is when excess sugar in the blood sticks to proteins in the blood, such as collagen and elastin. These damaging protein-sugar structures have been termed "the smoking gun" for almost every type of chronic disease, including premature aging and wrinkles. Glycation end products (AGEs) have been found at the sites of cancer, arthritis, and inflammation, as well as in the brain, where they are linked to Alzheimer's disease.[539-542]

Your Blood Sugar on Wheat

Today, popular theory is that grains in general are linked to blood sugar-related concerns and that they should be avoided,[3] yet the science suggests that whole grains are actually quite beneficial for stable blood sugar.[88, 120-123]

In a 2004 study in the journal *Diabetes Care*, researchers looked at data from over 2,800 people in relation to a condition called "metabolic syndrome," which is a condition that includes:

- Abdominal obesity ("sugar belly")
- High blood sugar
- Low levels of protective HDL cholesterol
- High triglycerides
- High blood pressure

Those who ate the highest amount of fiber from eating whole grains, including wheat, had a 38 percent lower rate of having metabolic syndrome. The group that ate the most processed and refined foods was found to be 141 percent more likely to have metabolic syndrome![120]

A balanced diet rich in whole, high-fiber foods including whole grains, legumes, vegetables, and fruits—foods that make up the Mediterranean diet[53]—have demonstrated over and over again to be key in reversing many of today's chronic health concerns.

A whole foods diet is also rich in essential minerals such as magnesium and calcium, which are natural antidotes to the sugar belly and the pre-diabetic epidemic we are now facing. In an 8-year study with over 40,000 participants, magnesium-rich whole grains, including wheat, were linked to a lower risk of developing type 2 diabetes. Researchers discovered the group that ate the whole grains as a source of their magnesium experienced a 31 percent reduction in type 2 diabetes. The group that ate a magnesium-rich diet without the whole grains only saw a 19 percent reduction in type 2 diabetes, which suggests that contrary to currently-trending popular belief,[3] whole grains like wheat may actually support healthy blood sugar levels.[121] Studies such as this suggest that wheat was not a problem for our digestion and health until we started mass-producing and over-processing it.

The grains you choose are critical in order to keep your blood sugar stable, weight down, and your heart healthy. Choosing organic, non-processed whole grains that are soaked, sprouted and fermented (sourdough) whenever possible that have the bran, germ, wheat kernel and endosperm still intact—with nothing added and nothing taken out—delivers the most vitamins, minerals and micronutrients which, as a natural food, supports optimal digestibility.[47]

Choosing ancient wheat grains whenever possible like einkorn, emmer, and Kamut® khorasan wheat are also important strategies. For example, 1 cup of modern wheat flour (white or whole) has about 95–100 grams of carbohydrates[543] compared to 60 grams in the einkorn wheat flour.[544] Einkorn wheat also has twice the fiber and 44 percent more protein,[543, 544] which significantly lowers the tendency for ancient wheats to increase insulin-stimulated fat storage or belly fat compared to modern wheat.[335] Ancient wheats like einkorn and emmer wheat also turn off genes that decrease sugar and fat metabolism, which may reduce the risk of type 2 diabetes.[545]

In our current culture of sugar excess, we should reduce the consumption of high glycemic foods whenever possible. There are many simple strategies to help lower the glycemic index of wheat and make it more digestible. In Chapter 7, I talked about how traditionally made sourdough breads create a low glycemic response as a result of the natural fermentation process.[338] Rye and spelt have also been shown to have a lower glycemic response than modern wheat and are great choices when sourdough or high quality whole wheat breads are not available.[545]

Let's not forget how nature intended us to consume most of our wheat. It was a fall-harvested grain to be eaten in the winter. Emerging science is suggesting that soil microbes that change from one season to the next also play a large part in digesting the foods that are naturally harvested in each season.[281, 285, 332]

Candida: A Sugar Dilemma

Candida albicans is a naturally-occurring fungus that lives in the intestinal tract. When it is allowed to overpopulate the gut as a result of a high-sugar diet, it can irritate and inflame the skin that lines the intestines, and cause a host of digestive-related concerns with a roster that parallels the symptoms of gluten and dairy intolerances.[546] Patients with candida symptoms typically report gas, bloating, abdominal pain, fatigue, swelling, brain fog, anxiety, depression, rashes and exacerbated food allergies.

In previous chapters, I have described the many ways the digestive system can go out of balance. Studies have confirmed that folks with Irritable Bowel Syndrome (IBS) and/or ulcers are most likely to experience candida overgrowth, along with all of the related symptoms.[547] Restoring the health of the intestinal skin and the lymphatic drainage around the intestines while turning on digestion is the most effective way to treat the source of a candida concern.

A diet of sweets, sugars, desserts, and simple carbs—as found in fast foods and processed foods—literally feeds candida overgrowth and disturbs the good bacteria in the gut.[548, 549]

Eating too much sugar is easy to do in our culture. Just one 12 ounce can of Coke has almost 10 teaspoons of added sugar,[550] and a Starbucks Grande

Vanilla Latte has 9 teaspoons.[551] Some sugars are often disguised as health foods. For example, a 15.2 ounce Naked Juice Green Machine is a healthy green drink, right? Did you know that it contains a whopping 13 teaspoons of sugar?[552]

Eating dried fruits is a very common snack that many folks consider healthy. However, consider this: A mango has about 4 teaspoons of sugar in the fresh fruit, but when you dry and eat the same weight as the whole mango, you are eating 19 teaspoons of sugar.

If you are experiencing the candida symptoms that I described above, and they are made significantly worse when you eat sugar, there is good chance you have a candida overgrowth.

To keep candida under control requires a thorough balancing of the digestive system and a repopulation of good bacteria. I prefer to begin this process with a regime of colonizing probiotics I described in Chapter 8, along with a candida-killing yeast called Saccharomyces boulardii.

Saccharomyces boulardii has been found to inhibit the growth of virulent candida as well as stop it from adhering to the intestinal bio-film wall. Saccharomyces has also been shown to reduce populations of other undesirable gut bacteria, which is why it is my go-to probiotic to knock out populations of unhealthy small or large intestinal bacteria and fungi like candida.[553]

Taking coconut oil, with its healthy antimicrobial properties, can also be very effective in preventing and treating candida overgrowth.[554]

The Price of Artificial Sweeteners

People who think they can have their sweetness without the calories or the sugar need to know there is no free lunch. Artificial sweeteners are major disruptors to digestive and intestinal health.

In one shocking study, researchers found that zero-calorie foods sweetened with artificial sweeteners like saccharin, sucralose, or aspartame all actually raised blood sugar levels![555]

After much investigation, scientists found that these artificial sweeteners actually harmed certain beneficial bacteria in the gut that were responsible for body weight and regulating blood sugar. Without these microbes, the sweetener was directed straight into the bloodstream, increasing blood sugar levels and body weight. As a result, there are many studies now linking the ingestion of artificial sweeteners to weight gain, likely due to the damage of the intestinal microbiome.[556]

We are beginning to see just how sensitive the body is to what it is fed and exposed to. And while the body is equipped to endure stress, toxins and bad foods, science is finding that the body and its microbiome maintain a sensitive, ever-changing and adaptive equilibrium in response to stressors from food and the environment.

Sugar Belly: An Early Warning Sign

Gaining weight around the midsection is most commonly a result of the insulin effect. Excess sugar in the blood will store as fat in and around the abdomen. This is the very first sign of a blood sugar disturbance and should be corrected with diet as early as possible. Yes, blood sugar will rise if we are eating processed wheat or any other processed food in excess. We have a blood sugar epidemic that is not caused by wheat, but rather a host of challenging lifestyle and dietary choices that are unique to each individual. Other than taking sugar out of the diet, which we should all be doing, there is no one-size-fits-all cure for the sugar belly.

New research is suggesting that fasting blood sugar levels that have been considered still within the "normal range" are now thought to be putting folks at a much higher risk for blood sugar-related issues such as weight gain (mostly around the belly), brain fog, fatigue, joint pain, cognitive and chronic health issues.[557-559]

Sadly, the "normal levels" for blood sugar levels used by most medical doctors allow blood sugars to become too high before suggesting dietary changes. Today, the normal ranges for first morning fasting blood sugars are between 70–99mg/dL. Often, doctors don't make recommendations until the sugars are well over 100, and that is just too late.

In one study, folks who had blood sugar levels just above 85mg/dL, well within the current normal range, had a 40 percent increased risk of dying from a heart attack or stroke.[557, 558] In another study, published in August of 2013 in the *New England Journal of Medicine*, study participants with blood sugar levels above 95mg/dL—again, still within what is commonly considered the normal range—had an increased risk for Alzheimer's.[560]

Troubleshooting Your Own "Sugar Belly"

Groundbreaking research at the Weizmann Institute of Science in Israel is in the process of monitoring the individual responses to high glycemic foods for over 1,000 patients. Based on the unique make-up of their microbiome, they are finding that everyone has a different blood sugar reaction to sugary foods. Some patients would get a blood sugar spike to sushi and grapes, but have no reaction to chocolate and ice cream. Some react to wheat and pasta and others do not. They are finding that it is all about the bugs in your gut. There are microbes that can digest wheat and some that can digest sugar. The capabilities of your intestinal microbes may have much to do with your food intolerances.

The good news, according to this study's research, is that the microbiome can change. As I have discussed, this all depends on the environment inside the gut and the health of the intestinal skin. Once this research is completed, these scientists hope to be able to recommend diets based on what your individual microbes can digest.[561]

If you have a sweet tooth, crave sugar, have extra weight around the hips or belly, or you're finding that you are becoming intolerant to foods you could once digest, consider monitoring your own blood sugar levels at home with an inexpensive over-the-counter glucometer. Nowadays, a blood sugar monitoring calculator can be purchased for $20–50, including test strips. They even have ones that plug right into your iPhone or Android. If your morning fasting (no food in the last 8–10 hours) blood sugar levels that fall consistently above the 100mg/dL range, find a holistic physician or nutritionist that will work with you to lower your levels and help prevent type 2 diabetes and other serious disorders as a result of consistently high blood sugar levels.

By using a blood sugar monitor, you can determine exactly what food is spiking your blood sugar. In the same way that your blood sugar might be spiked by your diet, it could also be spiked by stress or your lifestyle. For example, if you go out to dinner and have a glass of wine and dessert, you may wake up the next morning to find that your blood sugar level is much higher than normal. If you eat supper early and go to bed early, you may find the morning fasting blood sugar is back to normal. If you stay up late changing the world on your computer, the morning blood sugar level may rise. If you go to sleep stressed, the morning blood sugar may also be higher.

By self-testing your morning fasting blood sugar, you can begin to hone in on the cause of your blood sugar concerns, and then make the diet, lifestyle, daily routine, stress-management or exercise changes to nip a potentially very big problem in the bud. Don't wait for your annual visit to your doctor's office to be gently slapped on the wrist for overindulging.

You may also find that your sugar belly is related to blood sugar levels that are only slightly higher than normal or just on the high end of the normal range. If your morning fasting sugar levels are hovering around 100mg/dL, then we need to dig in and find out the cause. Getting your morning blood sugar numbers down into the 80s can take time. It took years for the blood sugar and digestive strength to get out of whack, so bringing it back into balance is more of a marathon mindset rather than a sprint.

Here are some of my top blood sugar-balancing strategies:

Start Checking Labels

Check the label on your favorite nutrition bar and you will find that it may be loaded with sugars. Remember, just because the sugar is made from date sugar, molasses, honey, dried mango, raisins, or fruit concentrates, doesn't mean it's healthy. Concentrated fruit sugars can spike blood sugar levels, triggering high insulin and a sugar belly.

The sugar content on the Nutrition Facts on a label will tell you the amount of sugar that is naturally occurring in that food, plus any additional sugar that is added in processing. You have to read the ingredient list to see if there are added sugars or sweeteners. You can also just do some comparisons. For example, a plain yogurt with nothing added may have only 6 grams of sugar, while a 6 ounce blueberry yogurt can have 25–30 grams of yogurt—a big difference!

Become a label reader! Do your best to avoid all sugars, sweeteners, and high-sugar content foods. Look for food labels with no added sugar or sweeteners and a sugar content of less than 6 grams per serving.

Get in the habit of comparing the sugar content in the breads, crackers, and dairy you purchase. Take, for example, in the Kavli cracker I mentioned in Chapter 7. There is "0" sugar and it tastes great. Kavli crackers do contain gluten, but in a non-processed form, with none of the "sugar belly" insulin-boosting effects.

Compare Kavli crackers to a Wheat Thin, which might have only 4 grams of sugar, but don't be fooled. Wheat Thins come with a litany of additives, preservatives, added sugar, and cooked oils, all of which make them much more difficult to digest.

Here are some of my favorite troubleshooting strategies for those hard-to-resolve blood sugar concerns. Check your morning blood sugars regularly during these trials so you can determine exactly which food or habit is raising the blood sugar. You can also use your blood sugar monitor to measure after-meal sugar spikes by taking your levels 1 and 2 hours after the meals (normal is below 125mg/dL 2 hours after the meal).

- Stop wheat for a week.
- Stop dairy for a week.
- Stop wheat and dairy for a week and stop them at night.
- Continued to test suspect foods by having them at dinner and checking blood sugar in the morning.
- Start exercising using my *Eat Wheat* Workout in Chapter 13 every day for a week.
- Cut out alcohol for a week.
- Go to bed before 10 p.m. for a week and get up with or before the sunrise.
- Don't eat carbs at night for a week.
- Stop eating after 6 p.m. for a week.

- Fast on water, or homemade Green Tonics (Chapter 10) 1 day each week for a month.
- Eat lightly (only 600 calories a day) for 2 days a week and eat normally the other 5 days for a month.

Grazing Versus Meals

Perhaps the biggest issue surrounding sugar belly and blood sugar concerns is the inability to burn fat as a natural source of fuel. As mass-produced, highly processed foods became the foundation of the American diet, we traded our ability to fuel ourselves with fat for a faster but not lasting, burning fuel—sugar. The result was the inability to make energy last and the need to eat more sugar, more often. To remedy it, grazing became the new norm.

 Tip: Find more on how to balance your blood sugar in my free *Blood Sugar Secrets to Health and Longevity eBook* at http://lifespa.com/blood-sugar-secrets-health-longevity/.

When the body is fed every 2–3 hours, it will burn fuel from those meals rather than its fat stores. So, instead of burning stored fat to make it from one meal to the next, the body becomes conditioned to be fed every 2–3 hours. A widely held belief is that if the meals are small, frequent, and healthy, the body won't store any fat from those meals and, in theory, have energy all day and never gain weight.

Here's the rub: When being fed every 2–3 hours, the body will not be encouraged to burn any of its stored long-lasting fat fuel for energy.[562-568] Why should the body bother digging out the fat stores to burn for energy when it is being fed all day long, every 2–3 hours? If, however, you only eat 2–3 meals a day and have ample time between meals, the body will be forced to burn stored fat between meals.

Remember, fat burning has a plethora of benefits beyond weight management. Fat is the most precious source of fuel for the body. It is the body's calm, non-emergency fuel. It burns slowly and steadily, providing energy for many hours straight. By contrast, sugar burns quickly. Sugar and carbohydrate fuels provide quick bursts of energy that often crash. Compared to sugar burning, fat burning delivers better energy, more stable moods, greater mental clarity, better sleep, less cravings, and of course, natural and permanent weight management.

To prove this point, I performed an unpublished pilot study in 2000 based on the principles in my book, *The 3-Season Diet*. We had the study group eat 3 meals a day with no snacks and measured weight loss and a host of psychological factors. Within 2 weeks, their moods, cravings, sleep, exhaustion after work, and fatigue were all significantly improved. Not only this, but they lost an average of 1.2 pounds per week for the 2-month study![569] For more information on balancing your weight, please download my free *Ayurvedic Weight Balancing eBook*[557] at http://lifespa.com/ayurvedic-weight-loss-ebook/.

How to Become a Better Fat Burner

When I was growing up, all the kids on my block had an early supper around 5:30 p.m. After supper, we played outside and then came in, washed up and went to bed. There were no bedtime snacks—the kitchen closed at 6 p.m. sharp. We would wake up and have breakfast around 7 a.m. and then walk 10 miles uphill to school in the snow. Just kidding, but that *was* 13 hours straight with no food! We slept through the night, fasting, and broke the fast with break-"fast." That means that every night, we reset fat metabolism. This allowed us to maintain normal blood sugar, stable moods, and overall greater health than what is created by the cultural habits today.

Eating breakfast, lunch and supper with no snacks will provide a natural fast between meals that will encourage fat metabolism.

What about Healthy Snacks?

If you have a healthy snack—like a carrot for instance—in between breakfast and lunch, you will burn fuel from the carrot. The carrot is healthy, but you will not burn any stored fat between those 2 meals. If you don't snack between lunch and supper, your body will be forced to burn stored fat to get you to supper without a blood sugar crash. From supper to breakfast is a critical time to burn fat, lose weight, detox, and reboot a stable nervous system to handle the stress of the next day… so you might want to rethink those midnight snacks.

Many folks have a major blood sugar crash between 3 p.m. and 6 p.m. They crave chocolate, a nap, chips or coffee. This blood sugar crash can be balanced with a shift in how we eat. Take time to have a large, relaxing breakfast—make that meal big enough to get you to lunch without the need of a snack. Then, make lunch the main meal of the day, and see how much food you need at lunch to get to supper without a snack. Make supper count, and see if you can eat nothing after supper until bedtime. Then, wake up and break the fast with breakfast. The key is to eat each meal slowly, calmly and joyfully.

Grazing is for Cows

Some experts say "grazing" (eating every 3 hours) will rev up your metabolism, control blood sugar, decrease hunger and create weight loss. These experts, however, are having a hard time finding any science to support their claims.

One of the main themes in support of eating 6 meals a day posits that it will keep the body's metabolism up, thus increasing thermogenesis (fat burning), resulting in weight loss. There are many studies disputing this notion. In 1997, the *British Journal of Nutrition* did a thorough review of all such related studies and found no evidence that eating 6 meals a day increases metabolism, thermogenesis, or weight loss.[570]

One of the other arguments behind the 6-meal-a-day plan is that if you eat 6 small healthy meals a day, the appetite and hunger at each meal will be less. This may help some dieters control hunger and calorie intake, but while the concept made many magazine covers, there appears to be little science to back this up.[571, 572]

Finally, perhaps the Holy Grail of "grazing" supporters is the claim that it helps balance blood sugar. If you open a medical textbook and look up "hypoglycemia," a condition of low blood sugar, you will see a recommendation to eat small meals throughout. It also suggests that once the blood sugar is brought back into balance, one would return to eating 3 regular meals.

True, eating frequent small meals a day will curb the highs and lows of the blood sugar and help folks feel more stable… in the short term. I have many patients who report initially feeling great on this plan: They start losing some weight, their anxiety levels, energy and cravings start improving. Soon, however, the body becomes dependent on eating every 2–3 hours. The ability to burn fat and make energy last disappears. Within 6 months, the results start to fade and the problems start coming back. They soon start feeling hungry all the time, the weight creeps back, and the anxiety and mood sensitivity can actually become worse.

Breaking the Grazing Habit

According to Victor Zammit, head of cell biochemistry at Hannah Research Institute in Ayr, Scotland, "If you eat only 3 meals a day, even high-glycemic ones, your insulin levels have time to even out."[573] Conversely, if you snack on high glycemic foods between meals, your insulin levels stay dangerously high.

In 2002, the New York Academy of Sciences came out with a report stating that grazing all day instead of eating meals may put you at risk for type 2 diabetes, heart disease, and stroke[574] for the same reasons I cited above. The only way we will reset our ability to burn fat as a stable source of fuel and digest well again is by eating less, less often. To accomplish this, we must first digest well. Most cultures around the world still eat 2–3 meals a day without snacking. For most Westerners who have become accustomed to snacking, having 3 meals a day will be a transition. Eating more than 3 meals a day has been linked to weight gain, angina, and a higher risk for chronic disease, so making this shift from grazing all day to 3 meals is important.[275] Give yourself some time to make this transition. You can even start with 4 meals a day to make the transition to 3 easier.

As you become a better fat burner, you will find that the amount of food you eat—and how frequently you eat it—will naturally decrease. I am recommending that your goal be 3 healthy, relaxed meals a day with no snacks. Once you accomplish that, don't be surprised if you find yourself only needing 2 large, relaxing and balanced meals each day with lots of water in between meals.

In India, there is an old saying:

1 meal a day is for a yogi
2 meals a day are for a bhogi (laborer)
3 meals a day are for a rhogi (sick person in a hospital)

They do not have a name for folks who graze all day as we do in the West. According to this saying, we are already sick eating 3!

Here are some tips to make the transition to 3 meals a day easier:
- Drink lots of water between each meal.
- When you eat: Relax, dine and enjoy your food.
- Make lunch the biggest meal of the day.
- Start with 4 meals a day, no snacks, and work down to 3.
- Make each meal count and try to make lunch the main meal.
- Avoid late night meals and start making supper smaller.
- Eat whole foods rather than processed foods.
- Strive for 50 grams of fiber per day. Fiber helps you feel satisfied. Remember, beans are one of the best high-fiber foods.
- Eat high-quality fat and protein with every meal.

Looking Ahead
With each seasonal change, nature harvests foods that encourage a natural detox of the body. In the next chapter, I will explore the strategies for a healthy and safe cleanse.

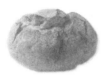

Chapter 12
LIVE TOXIN-FREE

T hroughout this book, I have been talking about the importance of a strong digestive system and how it is required to properly process and detoxify environmental pollutants, pesticides, preservatives and heavy metals. These toxins and pollutants are mostly fat-soluble, which means they have to be digested and then sent to the liver where they become water-soluble and then eliminated out of the body through either urine, feces, breath or sweat.

I have made the case that many Westerners have lost the ability to burn fat as a stable source of fuel and burn sugar-fuel instead. Without being a good fat burner, we lose the capacity to emulsify, process and detoxify toxic fats. As a result, these toxic fats find their way through the intestinal wall into the lymphatic channels. When these lymphatic channels become congested, fat-soluble toxins are redirected back to the liver. Here, over time, these toxins can overwhelm the liver and be recirculated back into the bloodstream where they are then ultimately deposited into the body's fat cells, or even more dangerously, into the arteries, heart or brain.[23-27]

Most of this book was dedicated to "teaching" us how to digest well, which enables us to protect ourselves from environmental toxicity and bad fats. What we haven't done yet is talk about detoxifying stored toxic fats that may have accumulated in the body's fat cells and brain for years.[23-27]

The concept of detoxification is by no means a new one. Traditional cultures have been employing detoxification techniques for thousands of years. While their environment was not nearly as polluted as ours, the digestive and lymphatic systems have always been vulnerable to irritation, inflammation and breakdown. When digestion breaks down, so does the ability to detoxify. Perhaps this is why we have so much extra intestinal skin. As we age, the health of the intestinal skin breaks down. There is much that can be done to preserve and protect the precious lining of the intestines.

I want to share with you a traditional detoxification therapy that is incredibly simple—it only takes 4 days, and it will detoxify undesirable fatty toxins from your fat cells while repairing the intestinal skin.[575] Many cleanses on the market go after the stored fat-soluble toxins by aggressively forcing them back into circulation to hopefully be flushed out of the body. Many cleanses are rough, exhausting endurance events that often leave folks quite debilitated. Somehow, traditional cultures understood how delicate the intestinal tract is and employed incredibly logical, kind, and gentle cleansing techniques to get the job done effectively and healthfully.

First of all, if you just pull all the fatty toxins out of storage and put them back into circulation and you do not address the reason why the body stored them in the first place, you might just be moving the toxins from one fat cell to another, and there's no guarantee that they will be escorted out of the body effectively. The digestive system must process these fatty toxins to be eliminated out of the body. If they have wound up in the fat, this is a strong indication that the digestive and detox pathways have broken down or are overwhelmed. To effectively and safely detox the body, it is important that we turn on the digestive and detox pathways *before* we start a detox. The cleanse I am about to teach you accomplishes both of these tasks.

This cleanse—which we call the *Short Home Cleanse*—employs the therapeutic principles of 2 foods we have already discussed in this book. They are the Ayurvedic superfood: kitchari, and the Ayurvedic superfat: Ghee. You can go back to Chapters 3 and 8 for a refresher on the benefits of these 2 foods.

In this cleanse, you will be taking small amounts of ghee (clarified butter) every morning for 4 consecutive days, during which time you will eat a completely fat-free diet. The preferred diet is kitchari, but I have supplied 2 other fat-free meal plans as options if eating kitchari alone is a bit too challenging.

Taking the morning ghee on an empty stomach while enjoying a totally nonfat diet during the day will ensure that the body continues to burn your body's fat throughout the day. If you include dietary fats during the day, the body will simply burn the fat that you ate for lunch and dinner instead of burning the stored fat and toxins lodged deeply in your fat cells and brain.

Studies suggest that ghee is an effective detox or chelating agent for eliminating environmental toxins.[575] The process of using ghee to remove fat-soluble toxins from the fat cells is called "lipophilic-mediated" detoxification, where the fat in ghee "likes" the toxic fats; it is attracted to them and attaches to them. This is how a healthy fat, like ghee, can be used to pull out unhealthy fats and/or toxins from your body.

In one study with 88 subjects, 48 of them consumed the ghee and kitchari as described above. The researchers measured 9 different environmental PCB toxins and eight pesticide toxins before and after the participants ate the ghee and kitchari.

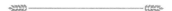

They measured a 46 percent decrease of PCBs, and a 56 percent decrease in pesticides!

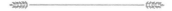

The study concluded that lipophilic-mediated detoxification may be effective in reducing body burdens of fat-soluble toxicants.[575]

Ghee is one of the highest food sources of butyric acid, and in this cleanse its job is to coat the intestines. In Chapter 3, I mentioned how the intestines have microbes that literally manufacture butyric acid and use this butyric acid as the primary source of energy and immunity for the cells of the intestinal wall while feeding many good intestinal bacteria.[196]

During the cleanse, the sequential increase of the morning dosage of ghee acts as a flush for the bile in the gallbladder and bile ducts. This increase in bile flow encourages and supports better fat metabolism as well as the production of HCl in the stomach, which is needed to break down wheat and dairy.

Eating kitchari is like eating medicinal baby food that supports a soothing repair of the intestinal skin while creating an environment for the beneficial bacteria that line the villi and lymphatic lacteals of the intestinal tract to proliferate. This provides a final seal and protective barrier for the intestinal tract that protects you from undesirable toxins and undigested proteins entering into the blood and lymph on the outside of the intestinal wall.

A few years ago, I was contacted by *Woman's World* magazine, asking if I could suggest a cleanse or detox program for their readers. I told them that I had a free eBook on my website called the *Short Home Cleanse eBook* and that it was a 41-page instruction manual of how to perform a cleanse at home that they could download.

Woman's World downloaded the free *Short Home Cleanse eBook*, gave it out to 40 of their readers as a small focus group, and said the results were phenomenal! People absolutely loved it. The cleansers reported losing up to 9 pounds in 4 days, felt more stable emotionally, decreased their cravings, and were digesting and eliminating way better than they had in years. Their focus group had such overwhelming success with the *Short Home Cleanse*, they wanted to write a feature cover story on the cleanse. The story was published on April 21, 2014, and they called it *The Colorado Diet Soup: Lose 9 lbs. in 4 days!*

I have provided an abbreviated version of the cleanse here for your convenience, but I also encourage you to read and download the free, full, 41-page version of the *Short Home Cleanse eBook* on my website at http://lifespa.com/cleansing/short-home-cleanse/. While there, I also invite you to look at our 2-week *Colorado Cleanse*, a more comprehensive home detox and digestive system reset that is easy and doable without having to take time away from work or your daily routine.

The 4-Day Short Home Cleanse (SHC)

Step One: Rehydration Therapy

One of the simplest and most important aspects of the SHC is to use purified, fresh water to rehydrate the digestive tract, as well as all the cells throughout the body. Please refer to Chapter 9, where I explain this 2-step approach in detail. In brief:

Hot Sips: Sip 1–3 sips of plain hot water from a thermos every 10–15 minutes throughout the day.

Daily Ounces: Drink 1/2 your ideal body weight in ounces of pure room temperature water everyday for 2 weeks.

Why Plain Water?

You may be wondering if you can swap your water out for lemon water, herbal tea, juice, carbonated water, coconut water, rice milk, or kombucha. During the SHC, it's important that the water for both our Hot Sips and Daily Ounces is plain and filtered. Plain water does not have to be digested as do the ingredients in other beverages.

I know it's a lot of water, so just do your best!

Step Two: Morning Ghee

Each morning, melt the prescribed teaspoons of ghee and drink on an empty stomach.

- Day 1—take 2 teaspoons of ghee
- Day 2—take 4 teaspoons of ghee
- Day 3—take 6 teaspoons of ghee
- Day 4—take 9 teaspoons of ghee

If it's difficult for you to drink the ghee straight, mix the melted ghee into 1/2 cup of warm almond, or coconut milk, or organic, vat-pasteurized and non-homogenized cow's milk. Drink the warmed mixture all at once. If needed, add a pinch of nutmeg, cinnamon, and/or cardamom for taste. Vegan alternatives for ghee are organic, cold-pressed, extra virgin olive or flax oil. Wait half an hour before drinking or eating anything after taking the Morning Ghee.

If nausea occurs, sip 1/2–1 cup of hot water with fresh lemon juice and grated ginger root. If nausea persists, do not increase the dose of ghee the next day—take the same dose or less, and be sure to eat breakfast (from your detox Meal Option of choice, below) half an hour after your Morning Ghee, even if you feel full, as this may help settle the stomach.

 Reminder: If your gallbladder has been removed, or you are experiencing trouble with your gallbladder, or have difficulty digesting fat, you may need to be on a modified protocol. If you do not have a gallbladder, you may substitute and use coconut oil instead of ghee, as coconut oil is easier to digest. If you have gallbladder issues or trouble digesting fats (nausea and indigestion after eating a fatty or fried meal), please stick with just 2 teaspoons of ghee or coconut oil each morning during the SHC, and do not increase the dosage.

Step Three: Eat 3 Meals a Day... and No Snacking

During the SHC, our goal is to teach our bodies how to enter into and maintain fat metabolism. One of the best ways to kick-start this process is to eat only 3 meals a day (along with the Morning Ghee), without snacking in between. This gives the body a chance to run out of its normal "go-to" fuel, which is carbohydrates, and switch to the calmer, more stable, detoxifying fuel of its own—stored fat. Sticking to 3 meals a day with no snacking turns you into a great fat burner!

The key to success with this is to make lunch your main and largest meal of the day. During lunch, take time to sit down, relax, and enjoy your meal without newspapers, books, listening to the news, watching screens or electronic devices—perhaps just some good company and calm conversation. This will help you leave the table satisfied. From there, you can aim for a lighter, smaller and earlier supper.

Eating this way requires some blood sugar stability. If 3 meals a day with no snacks is not possible for you yet, start with 4 meals, and work your way down to 3 at a comfortable pace. Don't stress too much about doing it perfectly, as stress can cause the body to store fat rather than burn it.

Foods to Avoid

To gain the most benefit from your cleanse, avoid these foods for the entire duration of the 4 days:

- Most important: Avoid all foods with fat, including oil, butter, avocado, nuts and seeds, dairy, fatty meat, and fish. (Except the ghee or oil substitute first thing in the morning.)
- Avoid bread, flatbread, crackers or any baked goods, as they slow down your detox.
- Avoid heavy foods (such as butter, yogurt, nuts, oils, cheese, and pizza).
- Avoid sprouts and curds (including tofu), pickles, and vinegar.
- Avoid soy (including tofu, tempeh, miso, and edamame).
- Avoid raw, uncooked vegetables and cold drinks, cold foods.
- Avoid white sugar, honey, alcohol, and recreational drugs, and caffeine.
- Avoid creamy (dairy) foods and spicy foods.

Step Four: Eat From One of 3 Meal Plans

Kitchari (also spelled: "khichadi," "kichari," or "khicharee") is your new best friend during the SHC, and a staple of each of the Meal Options.

Kitchari is an easy-to-prepare mixture of delicious organic long grain rice, split yellow mung beans and spices that is easy to prepare. Kitchari is high in protein and is extremely healthy for your digestive tract and intestinal mucosa. Find a recipe for kitchari in Appendix C.

Polydiet Meal Option

The Polydiet Meal Option is the most inclusive of different foods, and includes kitchari, steamed vegetables, oatmeal, salad, fruit, and protein. As this is the most diverse Meal Option available to you on the SHC, we recommend that everyone start with the Polydiet Meal Option.

The Polydiet is designed to be deeply nourishing even as your body clears toxins out of your fat cells and escorts them to your colon.

While the base of this Meal Option is still ideally kitchari, if you need a change, you can substitute a different small bean such as lentils, whole mung beans, or other large beans (like adzuki or black beans) and a different whole grain such as quinoa, millet, buckwheat, or amaranth, cooked into an easily digestible, porridge-like consistency.

To this kitchari base, you can add steamed vegetables, salad (raw seasonal vegetables), oatmeal, and/or other gluten-free grains. If you wish to eat raw fruit, Ayurveda recommends that you always eat them separately from other foods.

Additionally:

- Eat sweet fruits separately from sour fruits, and always eat melons separately.
- Only eat all-fruit meals if you have stable blood sugar, and ideally every other day at most.
- Breakfast is the best time for an all-fruit meal.

Duodiet Meal Option

The Duodiet Meal Option includes kitchari and steamed vegetables. If you feel ready for a more limited variety of foods, you can try eating just kitchari with some steamed vegetables or vegetable soup (homemade with vegetables that can be cooked with herbal seasonings and optionally pureed). While kitchari is preferred, alternative beans and grains are acceptable.

The Duodiet Meal Option is still nourishing in terms of giving you a multitude of minerals and vitamins, but it is slightly more rejuvenative to the liver and other organs as the fare is simpler and easier to digest than the Polydiet plan.

Monodiet Meal Option

The Monodiet Meal Option is comprised of kitchari only. To maximize your cleanse and reap the most benefits, eat only nonfat kitchari for your 3 meals each day. This will be incredibly healing to your digestive tract and extremely detoxifying. When you eat a Monodiet (comprised of 1 food), your body can focus the energy that normally goes towards digestion to cleansing and healing other systems. This meal plan is truly a transformative option for both your body's detox process and your psychological relationship to food.

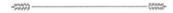

Troubleshooting the Short Home Cleanse
If, during the cleanse, you feel hungry, dizzy, moody, tired, nauseous, or uncomfortable, your blood sugar may be unstable.

If you experience these symptoms, add nonfat unadulterated non-processed whey protein powder concentrate (concentrates are less processed than isolates) in a shake, or a non-processed hemp seed protein powder if you are a vegetarian, or lean chicken or turkey to your meals—no matter what Meal Option you are following. While the key here is to avoid fat during the *Short Home Cleanse*, more protein may be needed to keep the blood sugar stable. If you are crashing in between meals, make sure you are on the Polydiet plan, have a nonfat snack that is high in protein, and plan to eat more protein at your next meal. Though the goal is not to snack, it can take some time to get the blood sugar to a balanced place where you can comfortably handle that much time between meals.

From my experience, it can take a few weeks to balance blood sugar, so there is no need to rush it during this cleanse. As I've mentioned, at no time during the cleanse do we want you to feel like you are starving or suffering, as it is also important that your nervous system is calm.

If this is your first time doing the *Short Home Cleanse*, I recommend that you begin with the Polydiet Meal Option and, in future cleanses, work your way to the Duodiet and Monodiet Meal Options.

Note: Straining during the SHC causes the body to store fat. Choose the Meal Option that is most comfortable in order to successfully reset your fat burning capability.

Step Five: Final Flush

On the evening of day 4, eat an early and light dinner. Wait 2 hours and then take a hot Epsom salt bath. If you cannot take a bath, take a hot shower and then rest with a hot water bottle on your abdomen for 10–15 minutes to warm the belly. Then, take your laxative.

Choose the laxative that is best for you:

- **For those with sensitive digestion** (*like regular heartburn and indigestion, loose stools, bowel irritation, gallbladder or liver issues*)
  - ◊ Drink 1 cup of senna tea (Traditional Medicinals Smooth Move tea works well).
  - ◊ Or drink 1 1/2 cups of room temperature or warm prune juice.
- **For those with healthy digestion**
  - ◊ Dissolve 1 tablespoon Epsom salts in 1 cup of water. Add 1 tablespoon of olive oil and 1 teaspoon of lemon juice. Drink the mixture.
- **For those with sluggish, hard or constipated bowels and strong digestion**
  - ◊ Dissolve 1 1/2 tablespoons of Epsom salt in 1 cup of water. Add 2 tablespoons of olive oil and 2 teaspoons of lemon juice. Drink the mixture.

You will likely experience a laxative effect within 1–15 hours after drinking the laxative (the average time is about 4–6 hours). If there was no laxative effect and you're still feeling strong, you can repeat the same laxative therapy on the fifth morning.

 Reminder: Check with your Medical Doctor before doing any laxative therapy.

Do not eat anything until the laxative effect has worn off. Sipping room temperature or warm water is fine. The cleanse is now over, but on day 5, break the cleanse gently with a soup or soupy hot cereal of well-cooked veggies and grains. My favorite first meal is baked sweet potatoes.

In the free 41-page *Short Home Cleanse eBook*, you will find detailed information about this cleanse along with herbal, lifestyle, exercise, yoga, breathing, and meditation recommendations to take this cleanse to the next level (http://lifespa.com/cleansing/short-home-cleanse/).

While the *Short Home Cleanse* is a quick detox and digestive reset, often the body needs more than 4 days to fully reset digestion and fully detox. As I mentioned before, to remedy this, I developed a 2-week cleanse and total digestive reset called the *Colorado Cleanse*. Learn more about our 2-week *Colorado Cleanse* at http://lifespa.com/coloradocleanse and enjoy the benefits of vibrant health and well-being!

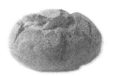

Chapter 13

THE *EAT WHEAT* WORKOUT

O ur bodies were meant to move, when they don't, bad things happen to the digestive system.

To start, the lymphatic system, which we now know is linked to the symptoms of wheat and dairy intolerance, depends on muscular contractions and exercise to flow. If the body does not get enough daily activity, the lymphatic system can become congested, as I have discussed earlier. Perhaps more critical is the congestion of the microscopic lymph vessels that drain toxins from the brain and central nervous system. Congestion here can affect how we think and disturb the function of the nervous system.

The benefits of exercise can be greatly enhanced when combined with correct breathing. How you breathe determines how well you will respond to stress, how well you will digest, the elasticity of the rib cage, and the movement of the lymphatic system.

My first book, *Body, Mind, and Sport*[576] compared the benefits of nose breathing exercise to mouth breathing exercise.[264] Let's look at some of the differences as they relate to digestion.

The Science behind Nose Breathing

In our research published in the *International Journal of Neuroscience,* nose breathing increased activation of the parasympathetic nervous system and quelled stimulation of the sympathetic (fight-or-flight) nervous system, during exercise. As I described earlier, parasympathetic (rest-and-digest) stimulation relaxes the body and engages the digestive system, while fight-or-flight stimulates the body and dials down digestive strength.

Imagine what would happen if you were startled by a bear in the woods. You would likely take a big, gasping, upper-chest breath through the mouth. Mouth breathing, according to our study, activates the fight-or-flight nervous system, which typically turns on in response to stress or an emergency.[264]

Mouth breathing fills up the upper lobes of the lungs where there is a predominance of fight-or-flight receptors. Nose breathing drives air through nasal turbinates, which are like mini-turbines that force air all the way into the lower lobes of the lungs, activating the parasympathetic receptors. Nose breathing also produces a significant amount of calm, meditative "alpha" brain waves compared to mouth breathing—making exercise less stressful and more enjoyable. Finally, nose breathing employs the entire rib cage to act as a lymphatic pump with every breath; that's about 26,000 times a day![264, 577, 578]

Take a Test Drive

Go for a walk and breathe deeply in and out through the nose. If you feel like you have to open your mouth to get enough air, you are going too fast. Slow down and catch your breath and start walking again at a slower pace while nose breathing.

While walking, count how many steps you take for each nasal inhale, and how many you take for each nasal exhale. Keep trying to take more steps for each breath. Gradually and painlessly, work up to taking 10 steps with each inhale and 10 steps with each exhale. The goal is to take longer, slower and deeper breaths, as this is what activates the parasympathetic nervous system.[579]

The goal is to establish full respiratory capacity which, depending on your body type, can reach as high as 20 steps during the inhale and 20 steps while exhaling. Just do the best you can, and watch your breathing improve.

This simple exercise is important. Most of us do not realize that the rib cage is constantly squeezing down on the heart and lungs. Each inhale requires quite a bit of muscular effort even to just take a breath, let alone breathe deeply into the lower lobes of the lungs. As a result, it is very common for folks to take shallow mouth breaths, 26,000 times a day, into the upper chest stress receptors which reinforce the message that life is an emergency.

Let's Talk About Yoga

Yoga is traditionally practiced with deep nasal breathing in order to create a yoga or "union" of the mind and body. The deep nasal breathing stills the mind while the yoga posture creates strength and flexibility in the body. The Sun Salutation is a series of yoga postures that is exceptional for helping to decongest the lymph and strengthen the digestive system.

The Sun Salutation is a series of flexion and extension postures that are coordinated with nose breathing inhalations and exhalations. As the body moves into extension, or leaning backwards, the breath is inhaled deeply through the nose. When the body flexes forward the air is exhaled completely. There are 6 inhale postures and 6 exhale postures.

While the chest is bending backwards and upwards during the inhalation, the diaphragm contracts downward as a way to pull air into the lower lobes of the lungs. As the chest is stretched up and the diaphragm contracts down, the two are stretched apart.

As the diaphragm contracts downward, it also pushes the abdomen down with it, including the stomach, liver and intestines. With the chest stretching upwards, this extends the diaphragm and adds a gentle stretch to the digestive organs as well.

The extension postures are immediately followed by a deep exhalation and flexion, or forward-bending posture, which squeezes the rib cage and abdomen together. During the exhale, the diaphragm relaxes, and the rib cage squeezes out the CO_2 from the lungs. Like an accordion, the body flexes forward and the rib cage and abdomen are pushed together, relaxing all the tension in the stomach and around the diaphragm.

The Sun Salutation focuses on the relationship between the stomach and rib cage, and delivers similar benefits as the stomach pulling exercise I described in Chapter 10. Many scientific studies have been conducted on the effects of this yoga sequence and suggest that the Sun Salutation increases parasympathetic activity, digestive strength and the ability to handle stress.[580-585]

Step One: Sun Salutation

This classic yoga sequence has numerous benefits that increase digestive strength and lymphatic flow.[580] To make this doable for everyone, I have included 3 different versions in Appendix D. There you will find diagrams for a classical version of the flow, as well as standing chair and seated chair versions, making the benefits of the Sun Salutation available for all levels of fitness. To reboot our digestive strength, we all have to move and breathe. Perform 5-10 minutes of one of the three versions of the sun salutation to start the *Eat Wheat* Workout.

Step Two: Begin Slowly and Breathe Deeply

For the next 5 minutes of your workout, start with very mild exercise. It could be a slow, rhythmic walk, jog, or bicycle ride. Begin to breathe long and deeply—as deeply in and out through the nose as you possibly can. Become aware of a very slight pause between your inhalation and the exhalation. Here we are exercising the lungs first, as the deep breathing requires much more exertion than the walk itself.

Step Three: Gently Increase Intensity

Slowly begin to walk, run, or ride faster. As you pick up the pace, try to maintain the same rhythm of the deep nasal breathing from Step Two, and try to maintain the slight pause between each nose breath. If the pause shortens as you speed up and you feel the need to breathe faster or open your mouth, you are going too fast. Slow down the pace and reset the original rhythm of your breath.

After resetting the original rhythm of your breath and reestablishing the slight pause between your breaths, begin to go faster again. Continue this for 15 minutes.[576]

Step Four: Move Like a Child

The next part of the *Eat Wheat* Workout requires 15–60 second sprints using deep nasal breathing. Choose how long the length of your sprint should be according to your fitness level. In between each sprint, enjoy a 1-minute slowdown or rest period. For example, if you are running on a track:

Sprint as fast as you can for 15 seconds (or however long your fitness level allows), then slow down to a walk for a minute. Then sprint for another 15 seconds and then slow down to a walk for a minute. Repeat this 2 more times, for a total of 4 rounds. As you become a better breather and more fit, you can extend the length of the sprint to a maximum of 60 seconds.

This is the lymph-moving part of the workout. It increases the intensity that is needed to fully contract and relax the rib cage and diaphragm. This step takes only 5–8 minutes.

The "sprint" doesn't have to be running. It can be jumping jacks, riding on a stationary bike, lifting cans of beans up and down as fast as you can over your head… you can be as creative as you like. The goal is to use your fast-twitch muscle fibers rather than the slow-twitch fibers that we use during yoga and hiking.

Step Five: Cool Down

Repeat the Sun Salutation for the next 5 minutes to complete the workout.

Why Exercise This Way?

Ask any healthy 10-year-old kid when was the last time they ran as fast as they could, and then ask the same of a 50-year-old. The 10-year-old would likely say, "I ran here!" The 50-year-old might say, "Hmm, it has been awhile. I think I might break!"

As we age, we slow down and mostly use our slow-twitch muscle fibers, but it is the fast-twitch muscles that help drive the sugar into the muscles and out of the bloodstream while flushing the lymphatic system.[586]

In one study, 1 hour after participants completed a 30-second sprint workout, growth hormone was measured to be 10 times higher than before they started the sprints. Maybe that's why kids do it—they thrive on growth hormone![587]

Human growth hormone, also known as HGH or the "youth hormone," decreases after 30 years of age and it is tied to aging. Exercise-induced HGH activation helps restore youthfulness and elasticity to the body. We are genetically mismatched to be sedentary. Sitting at a desk for hours at a stretch causes severe lymph drainage concerns that only make symptoms of wheat and dairy sensitivities more serious. Unfortunately, unless you are elderly, a stroll-paced walk isn't enough.

Fortunately, this simple yoga sequence and a fast-twitch exercise, while using deep nasal breathing, blends the best of both worlds. The combination of these 2 exercise techniques offers a wealth of benefits that target your digestive health and provide a pinch of the "fountain of youth" hormone.

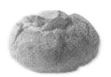

Chapter 14
MIND OVER BATTER

I've spent the majority of this book explaining the physical nature of good digestion and how to reverse the damage caused by a highly processed standard American diet. However, I'd be remiss if I didn't also address the critical importance of how the mind and emotions directly impact digestion, overall health and happiness. Our mind and body are inseparable, as we shall see with Charlie[7], a patient of mine who cured his gut and his mind, with his mind and his guts.

Charlie came to see me for gluten intolerance that he had been battling for years. Round after round of elimination diets left him with few foods that he could eat, and if he found something that helped him, it was short-lived. Once he found a plan, diet, pill, powder, or new miracle cure that gave him relief, it would only help him for a few short weeks.

In addition to his gluten sensitivity, he had been recently diagnosed with ulcerative colitis. He was completely exhausted with anxiety, panic attacks, and

---

7   All names of patients have been changed throughout this book to protect their privacy, and all patients have given permission to share the story of their health journey in this book.

unable to digest much of anything. He was dangerously underweight and rapidly losing more. His bowel movements were either nonexistent or explosive, and mucus made up the majority of his stool.

To help Charlie, I needed to start from scratch and reboot his digestive system. I knew the first thing I had to do was get him on the decoction recipe (described in Chapter 10) of slippery elm, licorice, and marshmallow root, along with amalaki to heal the intestinal skin and a colonizing probiotic to repopulate his gut with beneficial microbes.

After I gave him this initial protocol, I asked him what he thought was the cause of his chronic digestive problems. He told me without hesitation that it was emotional stress, explaining that his dad had put emotional pressure on him since childhood to perform and be the best at everything he did. Charlie never felt he was "good enough" for his Dad. Charlie said that he was lucky there was no physical abuse from his dad, but he had buried a lifetime of emotional pain from trying to be good enough. While he now lived far away from his dad, the mere thought of him caused his belly to tighten and start cramping.

The Mind-Body Connection

When treating the digestive system, we must take into consideration that the intestines are the first responder for the body's emotional stress—not the brain. Mental and emotional stress can cause significant damage and inflammation to the intestinal wall, and be lethal to the microbiology required to digest wheat and dairy. In the groundbreaking book *The Second Brain,* author Michael D. Gershon. M.D. discovered that 95 percent of the serotonin in the body, as well as most other brain neurotransmitters, are manufactured and stored in the intestinal tract—now called the "second brain."[390]

His research proved that we do indeed process our stress through the intestines, and the good bacteria that line the intestinal wall feel the stressors of the outside world and send that message to the brain through what is now called the "gut-brain axis." What the gut feels is quickly sent to the brain and, in short order, the whole body gets the message. If the messages are incessantly stressful, particularly in a child, the health of the good bacteria—and the ability for the nervous system to cope with such stress—will be challenged. In time, this can lead to serious intestinal health issues as well as adrenal and nervous system exhaustion, chronic fatigue, anxiety, and depression.[11, 13-15, 390, 396, 398, 399, 420, 428, 588]

Charlie literally had "gut feelings" as a young boy, in that his relationship with his dad did not feel emotionally safe. These gut feelings are being understood as part of the communication between the microbes and the brain. The subtle feelings and impressions that are conveyed by the gut are just now being understood by science.[400, 420]

The subtle perceptions of what the gut-brain relationship perceives has been linked to intuitive decision-making that researchers have confirmed as "gut feelings." When the intestinal skin and its microbes are healthy, the gut-brain and brain-gut relationship can activate higher cognitive and executive functions that researchers have found are in charge of our intuition.[420]

The higher intuitive functioning of the gut-brain axis is dependent on the health of the microbiome, which is in turn dependent on the integrity of the intestinal skin, upper digestive function, and the lymph vessels that surround the intestines. Optimal digestive and intestinal health is not only the key to eating wheat again, but, as it turns out, is linked to our emotions and intuitive decision-making as well.[220, 393, 399, 420, 428, 432, 433, 437]

When we think of the kind of daily stress Charlie was under as a child and how it impacted his intestinal health and his gut-brain axis, we have to take into consideration how this affected his mental, emotional, and overall physical health and consequently how his mental stress, in turn, impacted his digestive system.

Dopamine and Our Reward-Based Culture of "Never Enough"

Enduring childhood stress, as Charlie was forced to do, is not an uncommon experience. As children, we are all hardwired from birth to seek the approval of our parents. This ensures a feeling of safety and is linked to the survival of our species. Without the instinctive desire for approval from our parents and their consequent love, care, and protection, we may have dangerously wandered into the jungle and been attacked by a panther.

The problem is that most of us carry this desire for approval—as Charlie did from his dad—into adulthood. And unfortunately we rarely shed the need for emotional approval. Charlie was still scared of his dad because he still carried the hope for his approval. This desire for approval is chemically etched in our cells through the production of a reward hormone called dopamine. Whenever you get approval, win something, get good grades, fall in love, achieve something, get a "like" on Facebook, become a success, or accomplish most anything, you receive a "hit" of dopamine.

The problem with this hormone high is that it only lasts a short time. Once the reward-high wears off, we quickly find ourselves trying to fulfill the instinctive need for approval again by replacing it with the satisfaction from stimulants, including coffee, sugar, sex, money, fame, or we just go shopping—all of which stimulate the production of dopamine.[589]

While dopamine drives us to achieve great things; it also has a dark side—it is very addictive. Too much of this pleasure/reward hormone can breed excess. It can seduce us into overeating, a major cause of digestive issues and obesity.[590]

When it comes to dopamine, the old saying, "If a little is good, more is better" is not true. The key is in having a healthy balance of 2 naturally occurring hormones: Dopamine, and its polar opposite, oxytocin.

Oxytocin: The Loving, Giving Feel-Good Hormone

Oxytocin is a hormone that is linked to health and longevity, and unlike dopamine, where the receptors can become resistant to stimulation and require a more powerful stimulator, oxytocin receptors do not become resistant. Oxytocin is produced when you give, care for, love, touch, hold, hug, bond with, and nurture others.[591-595] Oxytocin has been shown to support cardiovascular health, brain function, digestive strength and much more.[391] The more you give, the more oxytocin is produced.[592, 596]

There is a catch, though. Only when you give without any expectations does it trigger the release of oxytocin.

The key is to bring these 2 hormones, dopamine and oxytocin, into balance. To do this, we must get in touch with our truth. As I have discussed in prior chapters, there is ample evidence to suggest that our microbes thrive in a positive environment and degenerate in a negative or stressful one. Giving fully, without any expectation of gaining something in return, triggers the release of oxytocin, which has a positive effect on health, longevity and your genes.[222, 399, 445-447, 597-599, 600-605]

Increasing Our Awareness and Transcending Our Old Patterns

Charlie had spent most of his life performing actions to obtain unachievable approval from his dad, and that lifelong habit had to be broken. I taught him how to meditate so he could become more self-aware and see the underlying emotional patterns that were actually driving him. With his newfound awareness and objectivity, he realized that as an adult, he was still acting out his childlike need for approval from his dad, and was able to release those patterns.

Like the lyrics in one of my favorite songs, he could "Let it go, let it go," because this behavior no longer served him; his father's approval wasn't necessary for his survival anymore. In fact, it was now compromising his survival. As soon as he became aware that he had a choice, he could "let it go."

As Charlie became more self-aware, he also realized that while his dad was a tyrant, he still loved him. So, Charlie started allowing himself to take some baby steps—acting upon his awareness—and began expressing his newly realized affection for his father.

Transforming old, unhealthy emotional behaviors, requires *action* in order to lay down new neural pathways in the brain that reinforce the production of oxytocin, rather than dopamine. For years, Charlie was *reacting* to the actions of his dad, and his dad was *reacting* to Charlie's. Neither of them was able to express their true feelings toward one another.

In taking his transformative action steps, Charlie started acting based on how *he* truly felt, rather than what he thought his dad would approve of. Charlie put his feelings into actions and regularly began expressing affection to his dad without any expectation of approval—or even the expectation to hear back from him. The key for Charlie was that he stopped caring about his dad's judgment, advice and criticism. He listened to him, but felt no obligation to perform. That simple shift freed him to act on his true feelings, which had been buried under years of emotional pressure. He was finally "doing Charlie" and he had stopped "doing" his dad.

Soon, Charlie started to feel better. He had fewer panic attacks and the emotional abdominal pain he felt when he thought of his dad was almost completely gone. He was making big strides with regards to his digestion and started reintroducing foods back into his diet that he had previously eliminated. After about 6 months of working with Charlie, he called me up and asked me if I thought it was okay for him to eat some pizza. I told him, "If you are considering eating pizza,"—a food that would have previously given him diarrhea for a week—"you must be feeling really good." I told him to give it a go. The last message I received from Charlie was that it was the best pizza he had ever eaten.

The mind is a powerful thing. In the end, our health, happiness and digestion is determined by the thoughts and actions that are initiated in the mind. In the first 6 years of life, 95 percent of the thoughts and actions we take are based on impressions we all experience. We carry these childlike emotions into adulthood and the stress, worries and fears keep pounding away at our gut wall, slowly weakening our digestion. These are called unconscious behaviors. To become conscious, we must first become aware of both the mind and the body. In this book, I have given you the foundation to bring the body and its digestion back into balance. Your next step is to become aware of the mind and its protective emotions, and then from this platform of a strong healthy body you can, like Charlie did, transform your gut and your mind, with your mind and some emotional guts! It does take some guts to take off your emotional armor and begin to love unconditionally. It is when we are able to replace dopamine with oxytocin and still be satisfied without the reward chemistry that we will finally be free.

I hope you are now ready to stop using restrictive diets to placate symptoms, and heal the root cause of your digestive disorders. Optimal digestion is your birthright and the key to a long and healthy life. I invite you to use the principles in this book to bring your digestion back into balance, break bread again, and avoid health problems before they ever arise. Bon appétit!

THANK YOU!

I hope you had fun reading about how you can start enjoying wheat and dairy again. Don't let reading this be the end of it! Not sure where to begin? Try the "Tips" throughout the book first, and then troubleshoort your specific digestive concern in Part II.

If you have a moment, please help others enjoy this book!

Review it! Help others choose what to read—tell them why you loved this book!

Authors live and die by reviews. It would mean a lot to me, if you learned something from this book, that you would leave a review. Amazon, iBooks, Nook, Goodreads, wherever it makes sense for you! If you do write a review, drop me an email at dr.douillard@lifespa.com and include a link to it, and if you like, request that I put you on my list of beta readers. You'll receive an invitation to review my next book ahead of the crowd.

Stay informed and receive the cutting-edge science on how we can continue to better digest wheat and dairy. Visit LifeSpa.com and sign up for my free *Video-Newsletter,* where I publish 3 articles and 1 video per week proving ancient wisdom with modern science. Let us become your resource for your natural health news!

JOHN DOUILLARD'S FREE
VIDEO-NEWSLETTER

Your News Source for Ayurveda and Natural Health

Check out the archives of 700+ original articles on natural health and Ayurvedic psychology at LifeSpa.com/articles

Love what you see? You can sign up to receive these cutting-edge health updates with an Ayurvedic twist in your inbox every week!
Sign up at LifeSpa.com/newsletter

REFERENCES

1. Fasano A, Sapone A, Zevallos V, Schuppan D. Nonceliac gluten sensitivity. Gastroenterology. 2015;148(6):1195-204.

2. MarketsandMarkets.com. Dairy Alternatives Market by Type (Soy milk, Almond milk, Rice milk, Others), Formulation (Plain sweetened, Plain unsweetened, Flavored sweetened, Flavored unsweetened), Application (Food & Beverages), & by Region - Global Forecast to 2020 October 2015. Available from: http://www.marketsandmarkets.com/Market-Reports/dairy-alternative-plant-milk-beverages-market-677.html.

3. Perlmutter DL, K. Grain Brain: The Surprising Truth about Wheat, Carbs, and Sugar—Your Brain's Silent Killers. New York: Little, Brown and Company; 2013.

4. Bloom GS. Amyloid-β and tau: the trigger and bullet in Alzheimer disease pathogenesis. JAMA neurology. 2014;71(4):505-8.

5. Louveau A, Smirnov I, Keyes TJ, Eccles JD, Rouhani SJ, Peske JD, Derecki NC, Castle D, Mandell JW, Lee KS. Structural and functional features of central nervous system lymphatic vessels. Nature. 2015.

6. Stetka B. Could Depression Be Caused By An Infection? 2015; October 25, 2015:[Available from: http://www.npr.org/sections/health-shots/2015/10/25/451169292/could-depression-be-caused-by-an-infection.

7. Canli T. Reconceptualizing major depressive disorder as an infectious disease. Biology of mood & anxiety disorders. 2014;4(1):10.

8. Benros ME, Waltoft BL, Nordentoft M, Østergaard SD, Eaton WW, Krogh J, Mortensen PB. Autoimmune diseases and severe infections as risk factors for mood disorders: a nationwide study. JAMA psychiatry. 2013;70(8):812-20.

9. Köhler O, Petersen L, Mors O, Gasse C. Inflammation and depression: combined use of selective serotonin reuptake inhibitors and NSAIDs or paracetamol and psychiatric outcomes. Brain and Behavior. 2015.

10. Wolfram-Gabel R. [Anatomy of the pelvic lymphatic system]. Cancer radiotherapie: journal de la Societe francaise de radiotherapie oncologique. 2013;17(5-6):549-52.

11. Brandtzaeg P. The mucosal immune system and its integration with the mammary glands. The Journal of pediatrics. 2010;156(2):S8-S15.

12. Harvey NL, Srinivasan RS, Dillard ME, Johnson NC, Witte MH, Boyd K, Sleeman MW, Oliver G. Lymphatic vascular defects promoted by Prox1 haploinsufficiency cause adult-onset obesity. Nature genetics. 2005;37(10):1072-81.

13. Vorvick LJubZ, David; Ogilvie, Isla; and A.D.A.M. Editorial Team; reviewed by. Circulation of Lymph. MedlinePlus. Updated 2014.

14. Streilein J. Skin-associated lymphoid tissue. Immunology series. 1988;46:73-96.

15. Cesta MF. Normal structure, function, and histology of mucosa-associated lymphoid tissue. Toxicologic pathology. 2006;34(5):599-608.

16. Choi I, Lee S, Hong Y-K. The new era of the lymphatic system: no longer secondary to the blood vascular system. Cold Spring Harbor perspectives in medicine. 2012;2(4):a006445.

17. Skobe M, Hawighorst T, Jackson DG, Prevo R, Janes L, Velasco P, Riccardi L, Alitalo K, Claffey K, Detmar M. Induction of tumor lymphangiogenesis by VEGF-C promotes breast cancer metastasis. Nature medicine. 2001;7(2):192-8.

18. Stacker SA, Caesar C, Baldwin ME, Thornton GE, Williams RA, Prevo R, Jackson DG, Nishikawa S-i, Kubo H, Achen MG. VEGF-D promotes the metastatic spread of tumor cells via the lymphatics. Nature medicine. 2001;7(2):186-91.

19. Das S, Skobe M. Lymphatic vessel activation in cancer. Annals of the New York Academy of Sciences. 2008;1131(1):235-41.

20. Wynn JG, Sponheimer M, Kimbel WH, Alemseged Z, Reed K, Bedaso ZK, Wilson JN. Diet of Australopithecus afarensis from the Pliocene Hadar formation, Ethiopia. Proceedings of the National Academy of Sciences. 2013;110(26):10495-500.

21. Cerling T. A Grassy Trend in Human Ancestors' Diets: U News Center; 2013. Available from: http://archive.unews.utah.edu/news_releases/a-grassy-trend-in-human-ancestors-diets/.

22. Revedin A, Aranguren, B., Becattini, R., Longo, L., Marconi, E., Lippi, M. M., Skakun, N., Sinitsyn, A., Spiridonova, E., & Svoboda, J. . Thirty thousand-year-old evidence of plant food processing. Proceedings of the National Academy of Sciences of the United States of America. 2010(107(44): 18815–18819). doi: http://doi.org/10.1073/pnas.1006993107.

23. Reynolds S, Aubele, T. The Skinny on Brain Fats Psychology Today2011. Available from: https://www.psychologytoday.com/blog/prime-your-gray-cells/201109/the-skinny-brain-fats.

24. Cojocaru M, Chicoş B. The Role of Heavy Metals in Autoimmunity. ROM J INTERN MED. 2014;53(3):189-91.

25. Caffo M, Caruso G, La Fata G, Barresi V, Visalli M, Venza M, Venza I. Heavy metals and epigenetic alterations in brain tumors. Current genomics. 2014;15(6):457-63.

26. Lang IA, Galloway TS, Scarlett A, Henley WE, Depledge M, Wallace RB, Melzer D. Association of urinary bisphenol A concentration with medical disorders and laboratory abnormalities in adults. Jama. 2008;300(11):1303-10.

27. Group EW. Body Burden: The Pollution in Newborns 2005. Available from: http://www.ewg.org/research/body-burden-pollution-newborns.

28. Whoriskey P. The U.S. government is poised to withdraw longstanding warnings about cholesterol 2015. Available from: https://www.washingtonpost.com/news/wonk/wp/2015/02/10/feds-poised-to-withdraw-longstanding-warnings-about-dietary-cholesterol/.

29. Foundation CD. What Is Gluten? : Celiac Disease Foundation; 2016. Available from: https://celiac.org/live-gluten-free/glutenfreediet/what-is-gluten/.

30. Foundation CD. Sources of Gluten: Celiac Disease Foundation; 2016. Available from: https://celiac.org/live-gluten-free/glutenfreediet/sources-of-gluten/.

31. Fenster CC, S. Gluten Free Whole Grains: Oldways Whole Grains Council; 2013. Available from: http://wholegrainscouncil.org/whole-grains-101/gluten-free-whole-grains/.

32. Kasarda DD. Can an increase in celiac disease be attributed to an increase in the gluten content of wheat as a consequence of wheat breeding? Journal of agricultural and food chemistry. 2013;61(6):1155-9.

33. Eitam D, Kislev M, Karty A, Bar-Yosef O. Experimental Barley Flour Production in 12,500-Year-Old Rock-Cut Mortars in Southwestern Asia. PloS one. 2015;10(7):e0133306.

34. Vigne J-D, Briois F, Zazzo A, Willcox G, Cucchi T, Thiébault S, Carrère I, Franel Y, Touquet R, Martin C. First wave of cultivators spread to Cyprus at least 10,600 y ago. Proceedings of the National Academy of Sciences. 2012;109(22):8445-9.

35.   Wisdom V. Gathering Wild Grains: Vital Wisdom; 2011. Available from: http://donmatesz.
       blogspot.com/2011/06/gathering-wild-grains.html.

36.   Council BoSaTfIDNR. Lost Crops of Africa: Volume I: Grains. Washington, C.C.: The National
       Academies Press; 1996.

37.   Rostami K, Hogg-Kollars S. Non-coeliac gluten sensitivity. BMJ. 2012;345:e7982.

38.   Magkos F, Arvaniti F, Zampelas A. Organic food: buying more safety or just peace of mind? A
       critical review of the literature. Critical reviews in food science and nutrition. 2006;46(1):23-56.

39.   Sinai ISoMaM. Children and Toxic Chemicals: Mount Sinai Hospital; 2016. Available from: http://
       www.mountsinai.org/patient-care/service-areas/children/areas-of-care/childrens-environmental-
       health-center/childrens-disease-and-the-environment/children-and-toxic-chemicals.

40.   Brown AC. Gluten sensitivity: problems of an emerging condition separate from celiac disease2012.

41.   Bureau USC. Population Clock: United States Census Bureau; 2016. Available from: http://census.
       gov.

42.   Diseases NIoDaDaK. Digestive Diseases Statistics for the United States National Institute of
       Diabetes and Digestive and Kidney Diseases: U.S. Department of Health and Human Services;
       2014. Available from: http://www.niddk.nih.gov/health-information/health-statistics/Pages/
       digestive-diseases-statistics-for-the-united-states.aspx.

43.   Gregorini A, Colomba M, Ellis HJ, Ciclitira PJ. Immunogenicity characterization of two ancient
       wheat α-gliadin peptides related to coeliac disease. Nutrients. 2009;1(2):276-90.

44.   Sofi F, Whittaker A, Cesari F, Gori A, Fiorillo C, Becatti M, Marotti I, Dinelli G, Casini A, Abbate
       R. Characterization of Khorasan wheat (Kamut) and impact of a replacement diet on cardiovascular
       risk factors: cross-over dietary intervention study. European journal of clinical nutrition.
       2013;67(2):190-5.

45.   Cooper R. Re-discovering ancient wheat varieties as functional foods. Journal of Traditional and
       Complementary Medicine. 2015.

46.   Lamacchia C, Camarca A, Picascia S, Di Luccia A, Gianfrani C. Cereal-based gluten-free food: How
       to reconcile nutritional and technological properties of wheat proteins with safety for celiac disease
       patients. Nutrients. 2014;6(2):575-90.

47.   Gunnars K. Why Modern Wheat is Worse Than Older Wheat: Authority Nutrition; 2014. Available
       from: http://authoritynutrition.com/modern-wheat-health-nightmare/.

48.   Azeke MA, Egielewa SJ, Eigbogbo MU, Ihimire IG. Effect of germination on the phytase activity,
       phytate and total phosphorus contents of rice (Oryza sativa), maize (Zea mays), millet (Panicum
       miliaceum), sorghum (Sorghum bicolor) and wheat (Triticum aestivum). Journal of food science and
       technology. 2011;48(6):724-9.

49.   Di Cagno R, Rizzello CG, De Angelis M, Cassone A, Giuliani G, Benedusi A, Limitone A,
       Surico RF, Gobbetti M. Use of selected sourdough strains of Lactobacillus for removing gluten
       and enhancing the nutritional properties of gluten-free bread. Journal of Food Protection*.
       2008;71(7):1491-5.

50.   Mofidi A, Ferraro ZM, Stewart KA, Tulk HM, Robinson LE, Duncan AM, Graham TE. The acute
       impact of ingestion of sourdough and whole-grain breads on blood glucose, insulin, and incretins in
       overweight and obese men. Journal of nutrition and metabolism. 2012;2012.

51.   Crane PK, Walker R, Hubbard RA, Li G, Nathan DM, Zheng H, Haneuse S, Craft S, Montine
       TJ, Kahn SE, McCormick W, McCurry SM, Bowen JD, Larson EB. Glucose Levels and Risk of
       Dementia: DrPerlmutter.com; 2013. Available from: http://www.drperlmutter.com/wp-content/
       uploads/2014/03/Glucose-Levels-and-Risk-of-Dementia.pdf.

52.   Hamblin J. This Is Your Brain on Gluten: TheAtlantic.com; 2013. Available from: http://www.
       theatlantic.com/health/archive/2013/12/this-is-your-brain-on-gluten/282550/.

53.   Gunnars K. Mediterranean Diet 101: A Meal Plan That Can Save Your Life: AuthorityNutrition.
       com; 2015. Available from: http://authoritynutrition.com/mediterranean-diet-meal-plan/.

54.   Solfrizzi V, Panza F, Frisardi V, Seripa D, Logroscino G, Imbimbo BP, Pilotto A. Diet and
       Alzheimer's disease risk factors or prevention: the current evidence2011.

55.   Wengreen H, Munger RG, Cutler A, Quach A, Bowles A, Corcoran C, Tschanz JT, Norton
       MC, Welsh-Bohmer KA. Prospective study of dietary approaches to stop hypertension–and
       Mediterranean-style dietary patterns and age-related cognitive change: the cache county study on
       memory, health and aging. The American journal of clinical nutrition. 2013:ajcn. 051276.

56.   Glazer H, Greer C, Barrios D, Ochner C, Galvin J, Isaacson R. Evidence on Diet Modification for Alzheimer's Disease and Mild Cognitive Impairment (P5. 224). Neurology. 2014;82(10 Supplement):P5. 224-P5.

57.   Lammers KM, Lu R, Brownley J, Lu B, Gerard C, Thomas K, Rallabhandi P, Shea-Donohue T, Tamiz A, Alkan S. Gliadin induces an increase in intestinal permeability and zonulin release by binding to the chemokine receptor CXCR3. Gastroenterology. 2008;135(1):194-204. e3.

58.   Neimark J. A Protein In The Gut May Explain Why Some Can't Stomach Gluten: NPR.org; 2015. Available from: http://www.npr.org/sections/thesalt/2015/12/09/459061317/a-protein-in-the-gut-may-explain-why-some-cant-stomach-gluten.

59.   Ji S. Opening Pandora's Bread Box: The Critical Role of Wheat Lectin in Human Disease: GreenMedInfo.com; 2016. Available from: http://www.greenmedinfo.com/page/opening-pandoras-bread-box-critical-role-wheat-lectin-human-disease.

60.   Grove H, Hollung K, Moldestad A, Færgestad EM, Uhlen AK. Proteome changes in wheat subjected to different nitrogen and sulfur fertilizations. Journal of agricultural and food chemistry. 2009;57(10):4250-8.

61.   Council WG. Research Sheds Ligth on Gluten Issues: WholeGrainsCouncil.org; 2012. Available from: http://wholegrainscouncil.org/newsroom/blog/2012/01/research-sheds-light-on-gluten-issues.

62.   Samsel A, Seneff S. Glyphosate, pathways to modern diseases II: Celiac sprue and gluten intolerance. Interdisciplinary toxicology. 2013;6(4):159-84.

63.   Agarwal R, Goel SK, Behari JR. Detoxification and antioxidant effects of curcumin in rats experimentally exposed to mercury. Journal of Applied Toxicology. 2010;30(5):457-68.

64.   Kislev ME, Weiss, Ehud, and Hartmann, Anat. Impetus for sowing and the beginning of agriculture:Ground collecting of wild cereals. PNAS. 2004;101(9).

65.   Rosenthal J. Integrative Nutrition. Austin, TX: Greenleaf Book Group LLC; 2007.

66.   Microbiology ASf. Humans Have Ten Times More Bacteria Than Human Cells: How Do Microbial Communities Affect Human Health? ScienceDaily. June 5, 2008.

67.   James JM, Sixbey JP, Helm RM, Bannon GA, Burks AW. Wheat α-amylase inhibitor: a second route of allergic sensitization. Journal of Allergy and Clinical Immunology. 1997;99(2):239-44.

68.   Gobbetti M, Rizzello CG, Di Cagno R, De Angelis M. Sourdough lactobacilli and celiac disease. Food Microbiology. 2007;24(2):187-96.

69.   Klingberg TD, Pedersen MH, Cencic A, Budde BB. Application of measurements of transepithelial electrical resistance of intestinal epithelial cell monolayers to evaluate probiotic activity. Applied and Environmental Microbiology. 2005;71(11):7528-30.

70.   Okada M, Kakehashi M. Effects of outdoor temperature on changes in physiological variables before and after lunch in healthy women. International journal of biometeorology. 2014;58(9):1973-81.

71.   Lindfors K, Blomqvist T, Juuti-Uusitalo K, Stenman S, Venäläinen J, Mäki M, Kaukinen K. Live probiotic Bifidobacterium lactis bacteria inhibit the toxic effects induced by wheat gliadin in epithelial cell culture. Clinical & Experimental Immunology. 2008;152(3):552-8.

72.   De Angelis M, Rizzello CG, Fasano A, Clemente MG, De Simone C, Silano M, De Vincenzi M, Losito I, Gobbetti M. VSL# 3 probiotic preparation has the capacity to hydrolyze gliadin polypeptides responsible for Celiac Sprue probiotics and gluten intolerance. Biochimica et Biophysica Acta (BBA)-Molecular Basis of Disease. 2006;1762(1):80-93.

73.   Press C. Western lifestyle may limit the diversity of bacteria in the gut. ScienceDaily. April 16, 2015.

74.   Doucleff M. How Modern Life Depletes Our Gut Microbes. NPRorg. 2015.

75.   Sarchett P. Is super-diverse Amazon microbiome something to strive for? New Scientist. 2015.

76.   Moroni AV, Dal Bello F, Arendt EK. Sourdough in gluten-free bread-making: an ancient technology to solve a novel issue? Food Microbiology. 2009;26(7):676-84.

77.   Rizzello CG, De Angelis M, Di Cagno R, Camarca A, Silano M, Losito I, De Vincenzi M, De Bari MD, Palmisano F, Maurano F. Highly efficient gluten degradation by lactobacilli and fungal proteases during food processing: new perspectives for celiac disease. Applied and environmental microbiology. 2007;73(14):4499-507.

78.   Nestle M. Animal v. plant foods in human diets and health: is the historical record unequivocal? Proceedings of the Nutrition Society. 1999;58(02):211-8.

79.   Carlson BA, Kingston JD. Docosahexaenoic acid biosynthesis and dietary contingency: Encephalization without aquatic constraint. American Journal of Human Biology. 2007;19(4):585-8.

80. O'Neil D. Patterns of Subsistence: Foraging: Anthro.palomar.edu; 2006. Available from: http://anthro.palomar.edu/subsistence/sub_2.htm.

81. Perry GH, Dominy NJ, Claw KG, Lee AS, Fiegler H, Redon R, Werner J, Villanea FA, Mountain JL, Misra R. Diet and the evolution of human amylase gene copy number variation. Nature genetics. 2007;39(10):1256-60.

82. McDougall J. For the Love of Grains: McDougall Newsletter; 2007. Available from: https://www.drmcdougall.com/misc/2008nl/jan/grains.htm.

83. Sabaté J. The contribution of vegetarian diets to health and disease: a paradigm shift? The American journal of clinical nutrition. 2003;78(3):502S-7S.

84. Sabaté J, editor. The contribution of vegetarian diets to human health. Forum of nutrition; 2002.

85. Sanz Y. Effects of a gluten-free diet on gut microbiota and immune function in healthy adult humans. Gut Microbes. 2010;1(3):135-7.

86. Reports C. 6 Truths About A Gluten Free Diet: Consumer Reports; 2014. Available from: http://www.consumerreports.org/cro/magazine/2015/01/will-a-gluten-free-diet-really-make-you-healthier/index.htm.

87. Liu S, Willett WC, Manson JE, Hu FB, Rosner B, Colditz G. Relation between changes in intakes of dietary fiber and grain products and changes in weight and development of obesity among middle-aged women. The American journal of clinical nutrition. 2003;78(5):920-7.

88. Foundation TGM. Whole Wheat: Whfoods.com; 2016. Available from: http://www.whfoods.com/genpage.php?tname=foodspice&dbid=66.

89. Harland JI, Garton LE. Whole-grain intake as a marker of healthy body weight and adiposity. Public health nutrition. 2008;11(06):554-63.

90. Good CK, Holschuh N, Albertson AM, Eldridge AL. Whole grain consumption and body mass index in adult women: an analysis of NHANES 1999-2000 and the USDA pyramid servings database. Journal of the American College of Nutrition. 2008;27(1):80-7.

91. O'Neil CE, Zanovec M, Cho SS, Nicklas TA. Whole grain and fiber consumption are associated with lower body weight measures in US adults: National Health and Nutrition Examination Survey 1999-2004. Nutrition research. 2010;30(12):815-22.

92. Giacco R, Della Pepa G, Luongo D, Riccardi G. Whole grain intake in relation to body weight: from epidemiological evidence to clinical trials. Nutrition, Metabolism and Cardiovascular Diseases. 2011;21(12):901-8.

93. Wu H, Flint AJ, Qi Q, van Dam RM, Sampson LA, Rimm EB, Holmes MD, Willett WC, Hu FB, Sun Q. Association Between Dietary Whole Grain Intake and Risk of Mortality: Two Large Prospective Studies in US Men and Women. JAMA internal medicine. 2015;175(3):373-84.

94. Nash DT, Slutzky AR. Gluten sensitivity: new epidemic or new myth? Proceedings (Baylor University Medical Center). 2014;27(4):377.

95. Fung TT, van Dam RM, Hankinson SE, Stampfer M, Willett WC, Hu FB. Low-carbohydrate diets and all-cause and cause-specific mortality: two cohort studies. Annals of internal medicine. 2010;153(5):289-98.

96. Lagiou P, Sandin S, Lof M, Trichopoulos D, Adami H-O, Weiderpass E. Low carbohydrate-high protein diet and incidence of cardiovascular diseases in Swedish women: prospective cohort study. Bmj. 2012;344:e4026.

97. Sieri S, Chiodini P, Agnoli C, Pala V, Berrino F, Trichopoulou A, Benetou V, Vasilopoulou E, Sánchez M-J, Chirlaque M-D. Dietary fat intake and development of specific breast cancer subtypes. Journal of the National Cancer Institute. 2014:dju068.

98. Wang X, Ouyang Y, Liu J, Zhu M, Zhao G, Bao W, Hu FB. Fruit and vegetable consumption and mortality from all causes, cardiovascular disease, and cancer: systematic review and dose-response meta-analysis of prospective cohort studies. bmj. 2014;349:g4490.

99. Mishra S, Xu J, Agarwal U, Gonzales J, Levin S, Barnard ND. A multicenter randomized controlled trial of a plant-based nutrition program to reduce body weight and cardiovascular risk in the corporate setting: the GEICO study. European journal of clinical nutrition. 2013;67(7):718-24.

100. Johansson I, Nilsson LM, Stegmayr B, Boman K, Hallmans G, Winkvist A. Associations among 25-year trends in diet, cholesterol and BMI from 140,000 observations in men and women in Northern Sweden. Nutr J. 2012;11(1):40.

101. Crane PK, Walker R, Hubbard RA, Li G, Nathan DM, Zheng H, Haneuse S, Craft S, Montine TJ, Kahn SE, McCormick W, McCurry SM, Bowen JD, Larson EB. Glucose Levels and

Risk of Dementia. New England Journal of Medicine. 2013;369(6):540-8. doi: doi:10.1056/NEJMoa1215740. PubMed PMID: 23924004.

102. Ehrlich SD. Constipation: University of Maryland Medical Center; 2013. Available from: http://umm.edu/health/medical/altmed/condition/constipation.

103. McIntosh GH, Noakes M, Royle PJ, Foster PR. Whole-grain rye and wheat foods and markers of bowel health in overweight middle-aged men. The American journal of clinical nutrition. 2003;77(4):967-74.

104. Nagel R. Living With Phytic Acid: Preparing Grains, Nuts, Seeds and Beans for Maximum Nutrition: The Weston A. Price Foundation; 2010. Available from: http://www.westonaprice.org/health-topics/living-with-phytic-acid/.

105. Slavin JL, Martini MC, Jacobs DR, Marquart L. Plausible mechanisms for the protectiveness of whole grains. The American journal of clinical nutrition. 1999;70(3):459s-63s.

106. Slavin J. Why whole grains are protective: biological mechanisms. Proceedings of the Nutrition Society. 2003;62(01):129-34.

107. Vucenik I, Shamsuddin AM. Protection against cancer by dietary IP6 and inositol. Nutrition and cancer. 2006;55(2):109-25.

108. Carney L. Phytic Acid in Grains? No Problem! : DrCarney.com; 2016. Available from: http://www.drcarney.com/topics/item/257-phytic-acid-in-grains-no-problem - .VpOD8kuft8O.

109. Tabak C, Wijga AH, de Meer G, Janssen NA, Brunekreef B, Smit HA. Diet and asthma in Dutch school children (ISAAC-2). Thorax. 2006;61(12):1048-53.

110. Perlmutter DaB, Bonnie J., Seeley, Randy J., Daniels, Stephen R., and D'Allesio, David A. Randomized Trial Comparing a Low-Carb Diet and a Calorie-Restricted, Low-Fat Diet on Body Weight and Cardiovascular Risk Factors in Healthy Women The Journal of Clinical Endocrinology & Metabolism: David Perlmutter MD; 2003. Available from: http://www.drperlmutter.com/study/randomized-trial-comparing-low-carb-diet-calorie-restricted-low-fat-diet-body-weight-cardiovascular-risk-factors-healthy-women/.

111. Anderson JW, Hanna TJ, Peng X, Kryscio RJ. Whole grain foods and heart disease risk. Journal of the American College of Nutrition. 2000;19(sup3):291S-9S.

112. Jensen MK, Koh-Banerjee P, Hu FB, Franz M, Sampson L, Grønbæk M, Rimm EB. Intakes of whole grains, bran, and germ and the risk of coronary heart disease in men. The American journal of clinical nutrition. 2004;80(6):1492-9.

113. Erkkilä AT, Herrington DM, Mozaffarian D, Lichtenstein AH. Cereal fiber and whole-grain intake are associated with reduced progression of coronary-artery atherosclerosis in postmenopausal women with coronary artery disease. American heart journal. 2005;150(1):94-101.

114. Johnsen NF, Hausner H, Olsen A, Tetens I, Christensen J, Knudsen KEB, Overvad K, Tjønneland A. Intake of whole grains and vegetables determines the plasma enterolactone concentration of Danish women. The Journal of nutrition. 2004;134(10):2691-7.

115. Djoussé L, Gaziano JM. Breakfast cereals and risk of heart failure in the physicians' health study I. Archives of internal medicine. 2007;167(19):2080-5.

116. Perlmutter D. Dietary Fat and Breast Cancer: David Perlmutter, MD; 2016. Available from: http://www.drperlmutter.com/dietary-fat-breast-cancer/.

117. Cade JE, Burley VJ, Greenwood DC. Dietary fibre and risk of breast cancer in the UK Women's Cohort Study. International journal of epidemiology. 2007;36(2):431-8.

118. Suzuki R, Rylander-Rudqvist T, Ye W, Saji S, Adlercreutz H, Wolk A. Dietary fiber intake and risk of postmenopausal breast cancer defined by estrogen and progesterone receptor status—a prospective cohort study among Swedish women. International Journal of Cancer. 2008;122(2):403-12.

119. Liu R. New finding may be key to ending confusion over link between fiber, colon cancer. American Institute for Cancer Research Press Release. 2004.

120. McKeown NM, Meigs JB, Liu S, Saltzman E, Wilson PW, Jacques PF. Carbohydrate nutrition, insulin resistance, and the prevalence of the metabolic syndrome in the Framingham Offspring Cohort. Diabetes care. 2004;27(2):538-46.

121. van Dam RM, Hu FB, Rosenberg L, Krishnan S, Palmer JR. Dietary calcium and magnesium, major food sources, and risk of type 2 diabetes in US black women. Diabetes care. 2006;29(10):2238-43.

122. Esmaillzadeh A, Mirmiran P, Azizi F. Whole-grain consumption and the metabolic syndrome: a favorable association in Tehranian adults. European journal of clinical nutrition. 2005;59(3):353-62.

123. Sahyoun NR, Jacques PF, Zhang XL, Juan W, McKeown NM. Whole-grain intake is inversely associated with the metabolic syndrome and mortality in older adults. The American journal of clinical nutrition. 2006;83(1):124-31.

124. Opie R, Itsiopoulos C, Parletta N, Sanchez-Villegas A, Akbaraly T, Ruusunen A, Jacka F. Dietary recommendations for the prevention of depression. Nutritional neuroscience. 2015.

125. Skarupski KA, Tangney C, Li H, Evans D, Morris M. Mediterranean diet and depressive symptoms among older adults over time. The journal of nutrition, health & aging. 2013;17(5):441-5.

126. Sánchez-Villegas A, Henríquez-Sánchez P, Ruiz-Canela M, Lahortiga F, Molero P, Toledo E, Martínez-González MA. A longitudinal analysis of diet quality scores and the risk of incident depression in the SUN Project. BMC medicine. 2015;13(1):1.

127. Knight A, Bryan J, Wilson C, Hodgson J, Murphy K. A randomised controlled intervention trial evaluating the efficacy of a Mediterranean dietary pattern on cognitive function and psychological wellbeing in healthy older adults: the MedLey study. BMC geriatrics. 2015;15(1):55.

128. Pusponegoro HD, Ismael S, Firmansyah A, Sastroasmoro S, Vandenplas Y. Gluten and casein supplementation does not increase symptoms in children with autism spectrum disorder. Acta Paediatrica. 2015;104(11):e500-e5.

129. Whiteley P. Nutritional management of (some) autism: a case for gluten-and casein-free diets? The Proceedings of the Nutrition Society. 2014:1-6.

130. Harrington J, Allen K. The clinician's guide to autism. Pediatrics in review/American Academy of Pediatrics. 2014;35(2):62-78; quiz

131. Potkin SG, Weinberger D, Kleinman J, Nasrallah H, Luchins D, Bigelow L, Linnoila M, Fischer S, Bjornsson T, Carman J. Wheat gluten challenge in schizophrenic patients. Am J Psychiatry. 1981;138(1208):11.

132. Lambert MT, Bjarnason I, Connelly J, Crow TJ, Johnstone E, Peters T, Smethurst P. Small intestine permeability in schizophrenia. The British Journal of Psychiatry. 1989;155(5):619-22.

133. Storms LH, Clopton JM, Wright C. Effects of gluten on schizophrenics. Archives of general psychiatry. 1982;39(3):323-7.

134. Jacka FN, Pasco JA, Mykletun A, Williams LJ, Hodge AM, O'Reilly SL, Nicholson GC, Kotowicz MA, Berk M. Association of Western and traditional diets with depression and anxiety in women. American Journal of Psychiatry. 2010;167(3):305-11.

135. Olveira C, Olveira G, Espildora F, Girón R-M, Vendrell M, Dorado A, Martínez-García M-Á. Mediterranean diet is associated on symptoms of depression and anxiety in patients with bronchiectasis. General hospital psychiatry. 2014;36(3):277-83.

136. Lee J, Pase M, Pipingas A, Raubenheimer J, Thurgood M, Villalon L, Macpherson H, Gibbs A, Scholey A. Switching to a 10-day Mediterranean-style diet improves mood and cardiovascular function in a controlled crossover study. Nutrition. 2015;31(5):647-52.

137. Choi HK. A prescription for lifestyle change in patients with hyperuricemia and gout. Current opinion in rheumatology. 2010;22(2):165-72.

138. Oliviero F, Spinella P, Fiocco U, Ramonda R, Sfriso P, Punzi L. How the Mediterranean diet and some of its components modulate inflammatory pathways in arthritis. Swiss medical weekly. 2014;145:w14190-w.

139. Olthof MR, van Vliet T, Boelsma E, Verhoef P. Low dose betaine supplementation leads to immediate and long term lowering of plasma homocysteine in healthy men and women. The Journal of nutrition. 2003;133(12):4135-8.

140. Detopoulou P, Panagiotakos DB, Antonopoulou S, Pitsavos C, Stefanadis C. Dietary choline and betaine intakes in relation to concentrations of inflammatory markers in healthy adults: the ATTICA study. The American journal of clinical nutrition. 2008;87(2):424-30.

141. Zeisel SH. Is there a new component of the Mediterranean diet that reduces inflammation? The American journal of clinical nutrition. 2008;87(2):277-8.

142. Vujkovic M, de Vries JH, Lindemans J, Macklon NS, van der Spek PJ, Steegers EA, Steegers-Theunissen RP. The preconception Mediterranean dietary pattern in couples undergoing in vitro fertilization/intracytoplasmic sperm injection treatment increases the chance of pregnancy. Fertility and sterility. 2010;94(6):2096-101.

143. Dhalwani NN, West J, Sultan AA, Ban L, Tata LJ. Women with celiac disease present with fertility problems no more often than women in the general population. Gastroenterology. 2014;147(6):1267-74. e1.

144. Shell ER. An Overreaction to Food Allergies: ScientificAmerican.com; 2015. Available from: http://www.scientificamerican.com/article/an-overreaction-to-food-allergies/.

145. Fleischer DM, Bock SA, Spears GC, Wilson CG, Miyazawa NK, Gleason MC, Gyorkos EA, Murphy JR, Atkins D, Leung DY. Oral food challenges in children with a diagnosis of food allergy. The Journal of pediatrics. 2011;158(4):578-83. e1.

146. Pediatrics FMNi. 'Shotgun' skin prick testing for food allergy held flawed: PM360online.com; 2014. Available from: https://www.pm360online.com/shotgun-skin-prick-testing-for-food-allergy-held-flawed/.

147. Imai T, Yanagida N, Ogata M, Komata T, Tomikawa M, Ebisawa M. The Skin Prick Test is Not Useful in the Diagnosis of the Immediate Type Food Allergy Tolerance Acquisition. Allergology International. 2014;63(2):205-10.

148. Education FAR. Skin Prick Tests: FoodAllergy.org; 2015. Available from: http://www.foodallergy.org/diagnosis-and-testing/skin-tests.

149. Shaw A, Davies G. Lactose intolerance: problems in diagnosis and treatment. Journal of clinical gastroenterology. 1999;28(3):208-16.

150. Hyman M. Dairy: 6 Reasons You Should Avoid It at all Costs: DrHyman.com; 2015. Available from: http://drhyman.com/blog/2010/06/24/dairy-6-reasons-you-should-avoid-it-at-all-costs-2/.

151. Kliem KE, Givens DI. Dairy products in the food chain: their impact on health. Annual review of food science and technology. 2011;2:21-36.

152. Huth P, DiRienzo D, Miller G. Major scientific advances with dairy foods in nutrition and health. Journal of Dairy Science. 2006;89(4):1207-21.

153. Fulgoni VL, Keast DR, Auestad N, Quann EE. Nutrients from dairy foods are difficult to replace in diets of Americans: food pattern modeling and an analyses of the National Health and Nutrition Examination Survey 2003-2006. Nutrition research. 2011;31(10):759-65.

154. Pittman G. Dairy products may lead to weight gain: ChicagoTribune.com; 2012. Available from: http://www.chicagotribune.com/lifestyles/health/sns-rt-us-dairy-productsbre88k124 20120921 story.html.

155. Chen M, Pan A, Malik VS, Hu FB. Effects of dairy intake on body weight and fat: a meta-analysis of randomized controlled trials. The American journal of clinical nutrition. 2012;96(4):735-47.

156. de Oliveira EP, Diegoli ACM, Corrente JE, McLellan KCP, Burini RC. The increase of dairy intake is the main dietary factor associated with reduction of body weight in overweight adults after lifestyle change program. Nutr Hosp. 2015;32(3):1042-9.

157. Zemel MB. The role of dairy foods in weight management. Journal of the American College of Nutrition. 2005;24(sup6):537S-46S.

158. Zemel MB. Mechanisms of dairy modulation of adiposity. The Journal of nutrition. 2003;133(1):252S-6S.

159. Zemel MB. Role of dietary calcium and dairy products in modulating adiposity. Lipids. 2003;38(2):139-46.

160. Committee TP. Foods and Arthritis: PCRM.org; No year listed. Available from: http://www.pcrm.org/health/health-topics/foods-and-arthritis.

161. Sköldstam L, Larsson L, Lindström FD. Effects of fasting and lactovegetarian diet on rheumatoid arthritis. Scandinavian journal of rheumatology. 1979;8(4):249-55.

162. Kedar E, Simkin PA. A perspective on diet and gout. Advances in chronic kidney disease. 2012;19(6):392-7.

163. Choi HK, Atkinson K, Karlson EW, Willett W, Curhan G. Purine-rich foods, dairy and protein intake, and the risk of gout in men. New England Journal of Medicine. 2004;350(11):1093-103.

164. Álvarez-Lario B, Alonso-Valdivielso J. HIPERURICEMIA Y GOTA; EL PAPEL DE LA DIETA. Nutrición Hospitalaria. 2014;29(n04):760-70.

165. Wolf M. Foods That Cause Brain Fog: Livestrong.com; 2013. Available from: http://www.livestrong.com/article/333669-foods-that-cause-brain-fog/.

166. Ozawa M, Ohara T, Ninomiya T, Hata J, Yoshida D, Mukai N, Nagata M, Uchida K, Shirota T, Kitazono T. Milk and dairy consumption and risk of dementia in an elderly Japanese population: the Hisayama Study. Journal of the American Geriatrics Society. 2014;62(7):1224-30.

167. Ogata S, Tanaka H, Omura K, Honda C, Hayakawa K, Group OTR. Association between intake of dairy products and short-term memory with and without adjustment for genetic and family environmental factors: A twin study. Clinical Nutrition. 2015.

168. Lee V. Which Foods Can Cause Nasal Congestion? : Livestrong.com; 2013. Available from: http://www.livestrong.com/article/30642-foods-can-cause-nasal-congestion/.
169. Wu□thrich B, Schmid A, Walther B, Sieber R. Milk consumption does not lead to mucus production or occurrence of asthma. Journal of the American college of nutrition. 2005;24(sup6):547S-55S.
170. Arney W, Pinnock C. The milk mucus belief: sensations associated with the belief and characteristics of believers. Appetite. 1993;20(1):53-60.
171. Pinnock C, Arney W. The milk-mucus belief: sensory analysis comparing cow's milk and a soy placebo. Appetite. 1993;20(1):61-70.
172. Grillo R. Seven Rasons Why We Have NOT 'Evolved' to Eat Meat: FreeFromHarm.org; 2012. Available from: http://freefromharm.org/animal-rights/seven-reasons-why-we-have-not-evolved-to-eat-meat/.
173. Evershed RP, Payne S, Sherratt AG, Copley MS, Coolidge J, Urem-Kotsu D, Kotsakis K, Özdoğan M, Özdoğan AE, Nieuwenhuyse O. Earliest date for milk use in the Near East and southeastern Europe linked to cattle herding. Nature. 2008;455(7212):528-31.
174. Curry A. 9,000-Year-Old Milk Cartons Found: DiscoverMagazine.com; 2008. Available from: http://discovermagazine.com/2009/jan/084.
175. Connor S. Stone age man drank milk, scientists find: Independent; 2003. Available from: http://www.independent.co.uk/news/science/stone-age-man-drank-milk-scientists-find-129153.html.
176. News B. Early man 'couldn't stomach milk': News.bbc.co.uk; 2007. Available from: http://news.bbc.co.uk/2/hi/health/6397001.stm.
177. Bulhões AC, Goldani HAS, Oliveira FS, Matte US, Mazzuca RB, Silveira TR. Correlation between lactose absorption and the C/T-13910 and G/A-22018 mutations of the lactase-phlorizin hydrolase (LCT) gene in adult-type hypolactasia. Brazilian Journal of Medical and Biological Research. 2007;40:1441-6.
178. No-Lactose. Lactose Intolerance: Geographical Distribution: SansLactose.com; No year listed. Available from: http://www.sanslactose.com/en/geographical-distribution/is/208.
179. McDougall JAM, Mary A. The McDougall Plan: New Century Publishers; 1983.
180. Holick MF, Chen TC. Vitamin D deficiency: a worldwide problem with health consequences. The American journal of clinical nutrition. 2008;87(4):1080S-6S.
181. Lipinski L. Milk: It Does a Body Good? : WestonAPrice.org; 2003. Available from: http://www.westonaprice.org/health-topics/milk-it-does-a-body-good/.
182. Ballentine R. Diet and Nutrition: A Holistic Approach. Honesdale, PA: The Himalayan International Institute; 1978.
183. Oster K, Oster, J., and Ross, D. . Immune Response to Bovine Xanthine Oxidase in Atherosclerotic Patients. American Laboratory. August 1974:p. 41-7.
184. Cohen R. Homogenized Milk: Rocket Fuel for Cancer: Health101.org; Year not listed. Available from: http://health101.org/art_milk_cancer_fuel.htm.
185. Levy TE. Optimal Nutrition for Optimal Health : The Real Truth about Eating Right for Weight Loss, Detoxification, Low Cholesterol, Better Digestion and Overall Well-Being. Blacklick, OH: McGraw-Hill Companies; 2001.
186. Oster KaR, D. The Presence of Ectopic Xanthine Oxidase in Atherosclerotic Plaques and Myocardial Tissues. Proceedings of the Society for Experimental Biology and Medicine. 1973.
187. Li W, Cen Y, Li X, Liao D. [Activity detection and immunohistochemistry study on xanthine oxidase in pathological scars]. Sichuan da xue xue bao Yi xue ban= Journal of Sichuan University Medical science edition. 2008;39(2):243-6.
188. Fallon S. Nourishing Traditions: The Cookbook That Challenges Politically Correct Nutrition and the Diet Dictocrats. Washington D.C.: New Trends Publishing; 2001.
189. Chen M, Sun Q, Giovannucci E, Mozaffarian D, Manson JE, Willett WC, Hu FB. Dairy consumption and risk of type 2 diabetes: 3 cohorts of US adults and an updated meta-analysis. BMC medicine. 2014;12(1):215.
190. Gunnars K. Saturated Fat: Good or Bad? : Authority Nutrition; 2015. Available from: http://authoritynutrition.com/saturated-fat-good-or-bad/.
191. Dhiman T, Anand G, Satter L, Pariza M. Conjugated linoleic acid content of milk from cows fed different diets. Journal of Dairy Science. 1999;82(10):2146-56.
192. Dilzer A, Park Y. Implication of conjugated linoleic acid (CLA) in human health. Critical reviews in food science and nutrition. 2012;52(6):488-513.

193. Gaullier J-M, Halse J, Høye K, Kristiansen K, Fagertun H, Vik H, Gudmundsen O. Conjugated linoleic acid supplementation for 1 y reduces body fat mass in healthy overweight humans. The American journal of clinical nutrition. 2004;79(6):1118-25.

194. Siri-Tarino PW, Sun Q, Hu FB, Krauss RM. Meta-analysis of prospective cohort studies evaluating the association of saturated fat with cardiovascular disease. The American journal of clinical nutrition. 2010:ajcn. 27725.

195. Koba K, Yanagita T. Health benefits of conjugated linoleic acid (CLA). Obesity research & clinical practice. 2014;8(6):e525-e32.

196. Araki Y, Andoh A, Takizawa J, Takizawa W, Fujiyama Y. Clostridium butyricum, a probiotic derivative, suppresses dextran sulfate sodium-induced experimental colitis in rats. International journal of molecular medicine. 2004;13(4):577-80.

197. Barcenilla A, Pryde SE, Martin JC, Duncan SH, Stewart CS, Henderson C, Flint HJ. Phylogenetic relationships of butyrate-producing bacteria from the human gut. Applied and environmental microbiology. 2000;66(4):1654-61.

198. Ghoddusi HB, Sherburn R. Preliminary study on the isolation of Clostridium butyricum strains from natural sources in the UK and screening the isolates for presence of the type E botulinal toxin gene. International journal of food microbiology. 2010;142(1):202-6.

199. Gao Z, Yin J, Zhang J, Ward RE, Martin RJ, Lefevre M, Cefalu WT, Ye J. Butyrate improves insulin sensitivity and increases energy expenditure in mice. Diabetes. 2009;58(7):1509-17.

200. Liebman B. Gut Myths: Nutrition Action Health Letter; 2013. Available from: http://www. readperiodicals.com/201301/2884546341.html.

201. Prevention NCDPOoD. NIH Consensus Development Conference: Lactose Intolerance and Health - Final Panel Statement: Consensus.nih.gov; 2010. Available from: https://consensus.nih.gov/2010/lactosestatement.htm.

202. Dixon JB. Mechanisms of chylomicron uptake into lacteals. Annals of the New York Academy of Sciences. 2010;1207(s1):E52-E7.

203. Guyton AH, John. Guyton and Hall Textbook of Medical Physiology, 12th ed.: Saunders; 2010.

204. Furness JB, Kunze WA, Clerc N. II. The intestine as a sensory organ: neural, endocrine, and immune responses. American Journal of Physiology-Gastrointestinal and Liver Physiology. 1999;277(5):G922-G8.

205. Vighi G, Marcucci F, Sensi L, Di Cara G, Frati F. Allergy and the gastrointestinal system. Clinical & Experimental Immunology. 2008;153(s1):3-6.

206. Chhabra RS. Intestinal absorption and metabolism of xenobiotics. Environmental health perspectives. 1979;33:61.

207. Stoven S, Murray JA, Marietta EV. Latest in vitro and in vivo models of celiac disease. Expert opinion on drug discovery. 2013;8(4):445-57.

208. Kohan AB, Yoder SM, Tso P. Using the lymphatics to study nutrient absorption and the secretion of gastrointestinal hormones. Physiology & behavior. 2011;105(1):82-8.

209. ProTheraInc.com. DPP-IV Enzymes: Clearing Up the Confusion 2010. Available from: https://protherainc.com/images/prod/UpdateArticles/2010_07_dppiv.asp.

210. Jessen NA, Munk ASF, Lundgaard I, Nedergaard M. The glymphatic system: a beginner's guide. Neurochemical research. 2015;40(12):2583-99.

211. Mendelsohn AR, Larrick JW. Sleep facilitates clearance of metabolites from the brain: glymphatic function in aging and neurodegenerative diseases. Rejuvenation research. 2013;16(6):518-23.

212. Canli T. Reconceptualizing major depressive disorder as an infectious disease. Biology of mood & anxiety disorders. 2014;4(1):1.

213. O'Donnell J, Ding F, Nedergaard M. Distinct functional states of astrocytes during sleep and wakefulness: Is norepinephrine the master regulator? Current sleep medicine reports. 2015;1(1):1-8.

214. UPMC CsHoPo. About the Small and Large Intestines CHP.edu: Children's Hospital of Pittsburgh of UPMC; 2015. Available from: http://www.chp.edu/our-services/transplant/intestine/education/about-small-large-intestines.

215. Miller MJ, McDole JR, Newberry RD. Microanatomy of the intestinal lymphatic system. Annals of the New York Academy of Sciences. 2010;1207(s1):E21-E8.

216. de Godoy JMP, Groggia MY, Ferro Laks L, Guerreiro de Godoy MdF. Intensive treatment of cellulite based on physiopathological principles. Dermatology research and practice. 2012;2012.

217. de Godoy JMP, de Godoy MdFG. Treatment of cellulite based on the hypothesis of a novel physiopathology. Clinical, cosmetic and investigational dermatology. 2011;4:55.

218. Liao S, von der Weid P, editors. Lymphatic system: An active pathway for immune protection. Seminars in cell & developmental biology; 2015: Elsevier.

219. Egawa G, Kabashima K. Skin as a peripheral lymphoid organ: revisiting the concept of skin-associated lymphoid tissues. Journal of Investigative Dermatology. 2011;131(11):2178-85.

220. Butler JE, Sinkora M. The enigma of the lower gut-associated lymphoid tissue (GALT). Journal of leukocyte biology. 2013;94(2):259-70.

221. Pabst R. [Lymphatic tissue of the nose (NALT) and larynx (LALT) in species comparison: human, rat, mouse]. Pneumologie (Stuttgart, Germany). 2010;64(7):445-6.

222. Bailey MT, Dowd SE, Galley JD, Hufnagle AR, Allen RG, Lyte M. Exposure to a social stressor alters the structure of the intestinal microbiota: implications for stressor-induced immunomodulation. Brain, behavior, and immunity. 2011;25(3):397-407.

223. Caminero A, Nistal E, Arias L, Vivas S, Comino I, Real A, Sousa C, de Morales JMR, Ferrero MA, Rodríguez-Aparicio LB. A gluten metabolism study in healthy individuals shows the presence of faecal glutenasic activity. European journal of nutrition. 2012;51(3):293-9.

224. Helmerhorst EJ, Zamakhchari M, Schuppan D, Oppenheim FG. Discovery of a novel and rich source of gluten-degrading microbial enzymes in the oral cavity. PloS one. 2010;5(10):e13264.

225. Finking G, Hanke H. Nikolaj Nikolajewitsch Anitschkow (1885–1964) established the cholesterol-fed rabbit as a model for atherosclerosis research. Atherosclerosis. 1997;135(1):1-7.

226. Crawford MA. The role of dietary fatty acids in biology: their place in the evolution of the human brain. Nutrition Reviews. 1992;50(4):3-11.

227. Prevention CfDCa. Diabetes Report Card 2014: Centers for Disease Control and Prevention; 2014. Available from: http://www.cdc.gov/diabetes/pdfs/library/diabetesreportcard2014.pdf.

228. Challem J. Stop Prediabetes Now: Wiley Press; 2007.

229. Berti C, Riso P, Monti LD, Porrini M. In vitro starch digestibility and in vivo glucose response of gluten–free foods and their gluten counterparts. European Journal of Nutrition. 2004;43(4):198-204.

230. Pellegrini N, Agostoni C. Nutritional aspects of gluten-free products. Journal of the Science of Food and Agriculture. 2015.

231. Cummins D. How American Food Makes Us Fat and Sick: PsychologyToday.com; 2013. Available from: https://www.psychologytoday.com/blog/good-thinking/201306/how-american-food-makes-us-fat-and-sick.

232. Rapin JR, Wiernsperger N. Possible links between intestinal permeablity and food processing: a potential therapeutic niche for glutamine. Clinics. 2010;65(6):635-43.

233. Liddle RA, Goldstein RB, Saxton J. Gallstone formation during weight-reduction dieting. Archives of internal medicine. 1989;149(8):1750-3.

234. Lewis TH. Gallbladder Disease Increasing and Trending Younger: Brattleboro Memorial Hospital; 2011. Available from: http://www.bmhvt.org/healthmatters/gallbladder-disease-increasing-and-trending-younger.

235. Siddiqui AA. Gallbladder and Biliary Tract: Merck Manual; 2015. Available from: http://www.merckmanuals.com/home/liver-and-gallbladder-disorders/biology-of-the-liver-and-gallbladder/gallbladder-and-biliary-tract.

236. Bowen R. The Gastrointestinal Barrier 2001; November 4, 2001:[Available from: http://www.vivo.colostate.edu/hbooks/pathphys/digestion/stomach/gibarrier.html.

237. Slyepchenko A, F Carvalho A, S Cha D, Kasper S, S McIntyre R. Gut emotions-mechanisms of action of probiotics as novel therapeutic targets for depression and anxiety disorders. CNS & Neurological Disorders-Drug Targets (Formerly Current Drug Targets-CNS & Neurological Disorders). 2014;13(10):1770-86.

238. Messaoudi M, Lalonde R, Violle N, Javelot H, Desor D, Nejdi A, Bisson J-F, Rougeot C, Pichelin M, Cazaubiel M. Assessment of psychotropic-like properties of a probiotic formulation (Lactobacillus helveticus R0052 and Bifidobacterium longum R0175) in rats and human subjects. British Journal of Nutrition. 2011;105(05):755-64.

239. Bravo JA, Forsythe P, Chew MV, Escaravage E, Savignac HM, Dinan TG, Bienenstock J, Cryan JF. Ingestion of Lactobacillus strain regulates emotional behavior and central GABA receptor

expression in a mouse via the vagus nerve. Proceedings of the National Academy of Sciences. 2011;108(38):16050-5.

240. Tillisch K, Labus J, Kilpatrick L, Jiang Z, Stains J, Ebrat B, Guyonnet D, Legrain–Raspaud S, Trotin B, Naliboff B. Consumption of fermented milk product with probiotic modulates brain activity. Gastroenterology. 2013;144(7):1394-401. e4.

241. Benton D, Williams C, Brown A. Impact of consuming a milk drink containing a probiotic on mood and cognition. European journal of clinical nutrition. 2007;61(3):355-61.

242. Rao AV, Bested AC, Beaulne TM, Katzman MA, Iorio C, Berardi JM, Logan AC. A randomized, double-blind, placebo-controlled pilot study of a probiotic in emotional symptoms of chronic fatigue syndrome. Gut Pathogens. 2009;1(1):1-6.

243. Dinan TG, Cryan JF. Regulation of the stress response by the gut microbiota: implications for psychoneuroendocrinology. Psychoneuroendocrinology. 2012;37(9):1369-78.

244. Desbonnet L, Garrett L, Clarke G, Bienenstock J, Dinan TG. The probiotic Bifidobacteria infantis: an assessment of potential antidepressant properties in the rat. Journal of psychiatric research. 2008;43(2):164-74.

245. Cani PD, Delzenne NM. Gut microflora as a target for energy and metabolic homeostasis. Current Opinion in Clinical Nutrition & Metabolic Care. 2007;10(6):729-34.

246. Crumeyrolle-Arias M, Jaglin M, Bruneau A, Vancassel S, Cardona A, Daugé V, Naudon L, Rabot S. Absence of the gut microbiota enhances anxiety-like behavior and neuroendocrine response to acute stress in rats. Psychoneuroendocrinology. 2014;42:207-17.

247. Bercik P, Verdu EF, Foster JA, Macri J, Potter M, Huang X, Malinowski P, Jackson W, Blennerhassett P, Neufeld KA. Chronic gastrointestinal inflammation induces anxiety-like behavior and alters central nervous system biochemistry in mice. Gastroenterology. 2010;139(6):2102-12. e1.

248. Dinan T, Cryan J. Melancholic microbes: a link between gut microbiota and depression? Neurogastroenterology & Motility. 2013;25(9):713-9.

249. Cryan JF, Dinan TG. Mind-altering microorganisms: the impact of the gut microbiota on brain and behaviour. Nature reviews neuroscience. 2012;13(10):701-12.

250. Forsythe P, Kunze WA. Voices from within: gut microbes and the CNS. Cellular and molecular life sciences. 2013;70(1):55-69.

251. Klarer M, Arnold M, Günther L, Winter C, Langhans W, Meyer U. Gut vagal afferents differentially modulate innate anxiety and learned fear. The Journal of Neuroscience. 2014;34(21):7067-76.

252. Christian LM, Galley JD, Hade EM, Schoppe-Sullivan S, Dush CK, Bailey MT. Gut microbiome composition is associated with temperament during early childhood. Brain, behavior, and immunity. 2015;45:118-27.

253. Grisanti R. Leaky Gut: Can This Be Destroying Your Health? : Functional Medicine University; 2016. Available from: http://www.functionalmedicineuniversity.com/public/Leaky-Gut.cfm.

254. Alexander J, Ganta VC, Jordan P, Witte MH. Gastrointestinal lymphatics in health and disease. Pathophysiology. 2010;17(4):315-35.

255. Giannelli V, Di Gregorio V, Iebba V, Giusto M, Schippa S, Merli M, Thalheimer U. Microbiota and the gut-liver axis: Bacterial translocation, inflammation and infection in cirrhosis. World journal of gastroenterology: WJG. 2014;20(45):16795.

256. Behar J. Physiology and pathophysiology of the biliary tract: The gallbladder and sphincter of Oddi—A review. ISRN Physiology. 2013;2013.

257. Lieberman D. The Story of the Human Body: Evolution, Health, and Disease: Pantheon; 2013.

258. A.D.A.M. Bile Duct Obstruction: NYTimes.com; 2012. Available from: http://www.nytimes.com/health/guides/disease/bile-duct-obstruction/overview.html.

259. Wiley. High-fat diet may cause changes in brain that lead to anxiety, depression. ScienceDaily. 2015.

260. Beck M. Emerging Type of Heartburn Defies Drugs, Diagnosis: The Wall Street Journal, wsj.com; 2012. Available from: http://www.wsj.com/articles/SB1000142412788732389470457811503169927 8010.

261. Richter JE, Katz, Philip O., Waring, J. Patrick. Introduction to GERD: International Foundation for Functional Gastrointestinal Disorders; 2010. Available from: http://www.aboutgerd.org/site/what-is-gerd/intro/.

262. Jones K. A Comparison of the Buffer Value of Bile and Pancreatic Juice Secreted Simultaneously. Experimental Biology and Medicine. 1931;28(6):567-8.

263. Qureshi WA. Hiatal Hernia 2016. Available from: http://emedicine.medscape.com/article/178393-overview.

264. Travis F, Blasdell K, Liptak R, Zisman S, Daley K, Douillard J. Invincible Athletics program: Aerobic exercise and performance without strain. International Journal of Neuroscience. 1996;85(3-4):301-8.

265. Travis F, Blasdell K, Liptak R, Zisman S, Daley K, Douillard J. Invincible Athletics Program: Exercise Without Stress. 1996.

266. Leak LV. Lymphatic removal of fluids and particles in the mammalian lung. Environmental health perspectives. 1980;35:55.

267. Froy O. Circadian rhythms, aging, and life span in mammals. Physiology. 2011;26(4):225-35.

268. Perkins A, Poole LB, Karplus PA. Tuning of peroxiredoxin catalysis for various physiological roles. Biochemistry. 2014;53(49):7693-705.

269. Cho C-S, Yoon HJ, Kim JY, Woo HA, Rhee SG. Circadian rhythm of hyperoxidized peroxiredoxin II is determined by hemoglobin autoxidation and the 20S proteasome in red blood cells. Proceedings of the National Academy of Sciences. 2014;111(33):12043-8.

270. Plikus MV, Van Spyk EN, Pham K, Geyfman M, Kumar V, Takahashi JS, Andersen B. The Circadian Clock in Skin Implications for Adult Stem Cells, Tissue Regeneration, Cancer, Aging, and Immunity. Journal of biological rhythms. 2015;30(3):163-82.

271. Thaiss CA, Zeevi D, Levy M, Zilberman-Schapira G, Suez J, Tengeler AC, Abramson L, Katz MN, Korem T, Zmora N. Transkingdom control of microbiota diurnal oscillations promotes metabolic homeostasis. Cell. 2014;159(3):514-29.

272. Orozco-Solis R, Ramadori G, Coppari R, Sassone-Corsi P. SIRT1 relays nutritional inputs to the circadian clock through the Sf1 neurons of the ventromedial hypothalamus. Endocrinology. 2015;156(6):2174-84.

273. Cadenas C, van de Sandt L, Edlund K, Lohr M, Hellwig B, Marchan R, Schmidt M, Rahnenführer J, Oster H, Hengstler JG. Loss of circadian clock gene expression is associated with tumor progression in breast cancer. Cell Cycle. 2014;13(20):3282-91.

274. Hu M-L, Yeh K-T, Lin P-M, Hsu C-M, Hsiao H-H, Liu Y-C, Lin HY-H, Lin S-F, Yang M-Y. Deregulated expression of circadian clock genes in gastric cancer. BMC gastroenterology. 2014;14(1):67.

275. Kahleova H, Belinova L, Malinska H, Oliyarnyk O, Trnovska J, Skop V, Kazdova L, Dezortova M, Hajek M, Tura A. Eating two larger meals a day (breakfast and lunch) is more effective than six smaller meals in a reduced-energy regimen for patients with type 2 diabetes: a randomised crossover study. Diabetologia. 2014;57(8):1552-60.

276. Center NLM. Calorie-restricting diets slow aging, study finds. ScienceDaily. 2014.

277. Jakubowicz D, Barnea M, Wainstein J, Froy O. High caloric intake at breakfast vs. dinner differentially influences weight loss of overweight and obese women. Obesity. 2013;21(12):2504-12.

278. Mazzotti DR, Guindalini C, dos Santos Moraes WA, Andersen ML, Cendoroglo MS, Ramos LR, Tufik S. Human longevity is associated with regular sleep patterns, maintenance of slow wave sleep, and favorable lipid profile. Frontiers in aging neuroscience. 2014;6.

279. Vege SS, Locke GR, Weaver AL, Farmer SA, Melton LJ, Talley NJ, editors. Functional gastrointestinal disorders among people with sleep disturbances: a population-based study. Mayo Clinic Proceedings; 2004: Elsevier.

280. Kim HI, Jung S, Choi JY, Kim S-E, Jung H-K, Shim K-N, Yoo K. Impact of shiftwork on irritable bowel syndrome and functional dyspepsia. Journal of Korean medical science. 2013;28(3):431-7.

281. Davenport ER, Mizrahi-Man O, Michelini K, Barreiro LB, Ober C, Gilad Y. Seasonal variation in human gut microbiome composition. PloS one. 2014;9(3):e90731.

282. Haskell DG. The Forest Unseen: A Year's Watch In Nature: Penguin Books; 2012.

283. Rahmathulla V, Suresh H. Seasonal variation in food consumption, assimilation, and conversion efficiency of Indian bivoltine hybrid silkworm, Bombyx mori. Journal of Insect Science. 2012;12(1):82.

284. Buehner KP, Anand S, Garcia A. Prevalence of thermoduric bacteria and spores on 10 Midwest dairy farms. Journal of dairy science. 2014;97(11):6777-84.

285. Bowers RM, Clements N, Emerson JB, Wiedinmyer C, Hannigan MP, Fierer N. Seasonal variability in bacterial and fungal diversity of the near-surface atmosphere. Environmental science & technology. 2013;47(21):12097-106.

286. Kiernan B. Grass Fed versus Corn Fed: You Are What Your Food Eats: Global AgInvesting; 2012. Available from: http://www.globalaginvesting.com/news/blogdetail?contentid=1479.

287. Zhang J, Guo Z, Lim AAQ, Zheng Y, Koh EY, Ho D, Qiao J, Huo D, Hou Q, Huang W. Mongolians core gut microbiota and its correlation with seasonal dietary changes. Scientific reports. 2014;4.

288. Basulto D. The secret to treating your allergies may lie in your stomach: The Washington Post; 2014. Available from: https://www.washingtonpost.com/news/innovations/wp/2014/04/17/the-secret-to-treating-your-allergies-may-lie-in-your-stomach/.

289. Summa KC, Turek FW. The Clocks within Us. Scientific American. 2015;312(2):50-5.

290. University AFoTA. Eating a big breakfast fights obesity and disease: ScienceDaily; 2013. Available from: http://www.sciencedaily.com/releases/2013/08/130805131011.htm.

291. Yoshizaki T, Tada Y, Hida A, Sunami A, Yokoyama Y, Yasuda J, Nakai A, Togo F, Kawano Y. Effects of feeding schedule changes on the circadian phase of the cardiac autonomic nervous system and serum lipid levels. European journal of applied physiology. 2013;113(10):2603-11.

292. Harmon K. Breakfast Is the Most Important Meal for Dieters. Scientific American. 2013.

293. Kobayashi F, Ogata H, Omi N, Nagasaka S, Yamaguchi S, Hibi M, Tokuyama K. Effect of breakfast skipping on diurnal variation of energy metabolism and blood glucose. Obesity research & clinical practice. 2014;8(3):e249-e57.

294. Douillard J. The 3-Season Diet. New York: Harmony Books; 2000.

295. Goodspeed D, Liu JD, Chehab EW, Sheng Z, Francisco M, Kliebenstein DJ, Braam J. Postharvest circadian entrainment enhances crop pest resistance and phytochemical cycling. Current Biology. 2013;23(13):1235-41.

296. Braam JaF, Ira. Vegetables Respond to a Daily Clock, Even After Harvest: NPR; 2013. Available from: http://www.npr.org/2013/06/21/194230818/vegetables-respond-to-a-daily-clock-even-after-harvest.

297. Mamerow MM, Mettler JA, English KL, Casperson SL, Arentson-Lantz E, Sheffield Moore M, Layman DK, Paddon-Jones D. Dietary protein distribution positively influences 24-h muscle protein synthesis in healthy adults. The Journal of nutrition. 2014;144(6):876-80.

298. Jung CM, Khalsa SBS, Scheer FA, Cajochen C, Lockley SW, Czeisler CA, Wright KP. Acute effects of bright light exposure on cortisol levels. Journal of biological rhythms. 2010;25(3):208-16.

299. Center UoRM. To Sleep, Perchance to Clean: University of Rochester Medical Center; 2013. Available from: https://www.urmc.rochester.edu/news/story/3956/to-sleep-perchance-to-clean.aspx.

300. Merkulov Y, Pyatkov A, Merkulova D. [Work with night shift as a factor dysregulation of autonomic nervous system of locomotive drivers]. Patologicheskaia fiziologiia i eksperimental'naia terapiia. 2012(1):75-80.

301. Buijs RM, Escobar C, Swaab DF. The circadian system and the balance of the autonomic nervous system. Handb Clin Neurol. 2013;117:173-91.

302. Schwartz JR, Roth T. Neurophysiology of sleep and wakefulness: basic science and clinical implications. Current neuropharmacology. 2008;6(4):367.

303. Sasaki-Otomaru A, Sakuma Y, Mochizuki Y, Ishida S, Kanoya Y, Sato C. Effect of regular gum chewing on levels of anxiety, mood, and fatigue in healthy young adults. Clinical practice and epidemiology in mental health: CP & EMH. 2011;7:133.

304. Hirano Y, Onozuka M. Chewing and attention: a positive effect on sustained attention. BioMed Research International. 2015;2015.

305. Shao Q, Chin K-V. Survey of American food trends and the growing obesity epidemic. Nutrition research and practice. 2011;5(3):253-9.

306. Ladabaum U, Mannalithara A, Myer PA, Singh G. Obesity, abdominal obesity, physical activity, and caloric intake in US adults: 1988 to 2010. The American journal of medicine. 2014;127(8):717-27. e12.

307. Young LR, Nestle M. The contribution of expanding portion sizes to the US obesity epidemic. American journal of public health. 2002;92(2):246-9.

308. Corporation S. Company Information: Starbucks Corporation; 2016. Available from: http://www.starbucks.com/about-us/company-information.

309. Corporation S. Frappuccino Turns 20: The Story behind Starbucks Beloved Beverage: Starbucks Corporation; 2015. Available from: https://news.starbucks.com/news/frappuccino-turns-20.

310. Corporation S. Caramel Cocoa Cluster Frappuccino® Blended Coffee: Starbucks Corporation; 2016. Available from: http://www.starbucks.com/menu/drinks/frappuccino-blended-beverages/caramel-cocoa-cluster-frappuccino-blended-beverage, http://www.starbucks.com/menu/drinks/frappuccino-blended-beverages/caramel-cocoa-cluster-frappuccino-blended-beverage - size=11050788&milk=67&whip=125.

311. McCay C, Crowell MF, Maynard L. The effect of retarded growth upon the length of life span and upon the ultimate body size. J nutr. 1935;10(1):63-79.

312. Mattison JA, Roth GS, Beasley TM, Tilmont EM, Handy AM, Herbert RL, Longo DL, Allison DB, Young JE, Bryant M. Impact of caloric restriction on health and survival in rhesus monkeys from the NIA study. Nature. 2012.

313. Everitt AV, COUTEUR L, DAVID G. Life extension by calorie restriction in humans. Annals of the New York Academy of Sciences. 2007;1114(1):428-33.

314. Calnan D, Brunet A. The foxo code. Oncogene. 2008;27(16):2276-88.

315. McGlothin P, Averill M. How Glucose Mediates Life And Death By Turning Genes On And Off. Life Extension Magazine. 2014;20(2):50-5.

316. McCarthy M. Higher sugar intake linked to raised risk of cardiovascular mortality, study finds. Bmj. 2014;348.

317. Yang Q, Zhang Z, Gregg EW, Flanders WD, Merritt R, Hu FB. Added sugar intake and cardiovascular diseases mortality among US adults. JAMA internal medicine. 2014;174(4):516-24.

318. Messina V. Nutritional and health benefits of dried beans. The American journal of clinical nutrition. 2014;100(Supplement 1):437S-42S.

319. Bouchenak M, Lamri-Senhadji M. Nutritional quality of legumes, and their role in cardiometabolic risk prevention: a review. Journal of medicinal food. 2013;16(3):185-98.

320. Nilsson A, Johansson E, Ekstrom L, Bjorck I. Effects of a brown beans evening meal on metabolic risk markers and appetite regulating hormones at a subsequent standardized breakfast: a randomized cross-over study. PloS one. 2013;8(4):e59985.

321. Gandhi GR, Vanlalhruaia P, Stalin A, Irudayaraj SS, Ignacimuthu S, Paulraj MG. Polyphenols-rich Cyamopsis tetragonoloba (L.) Taub. beans show hypoglycemic and β-cells protective effects in type 2 diabetic rats. Food and Chemical Toxicology. 2014;66:358-65.

322. Luhovyy BL, Mollard RC, Panahi S, Nunez MF, Cho F, Anderson GH. Canned Navy Bean Consumption Reduces Metabolic Risk Factors Associated with Obesity. Canadian Journal of Dietetic Practice and Research. 2015;76(1):33-7.

323. Vij VA, Joshi AS. Effect of 'water induced thermogenesis' on body weight, body mass index and body composition of overweight subjects. Journal of clinical and diagnostic research: JCDR. 2013;7(9):1894.

324. Shantha M. Sleep loss and circadian disruption in shift work: health burden and management. The Medical journal of Australia. 2013;199(8):11-5.

325. Banerjee R, Hazra S, Ghosh AK, Mondal AC. Chronic administration of bacopa monniera increases BDNF protein and mRNA expressions: a study in chronic unpredictable stress induced animal model of depression. Psychiatry investigation. 2014;11(3):297-306.

326. Science.gov. Bacopa monniera: Science.gov; Year unlisted. Available from: http://www.science.gov/topicpages/b/bacopa+monniera+linn.html.

327. Konar A, Shah N, Singh R, Saxena N, Kaul SC, Wadhwa R, Thakur MK. Protective role of Ashwagandha leaf extract and its component withanone on scopolamine-induced changes in the brain and brain-derived cells. PloS one. 2011;6(11):e27265.

328. Hucklenbroich J, Klein R, Neumaier B, Graf R, Fink GR, Schroeter M, Rueger MA. Aromatic-turmerone induces neural stem cell proliferation in vitro and in vivo. Stem cell research & therapy. 2014;5(4):100.

329. Bazian NC. Could curry spice boost brain cell repair?2014.

330. Yu Y, Wu S, Li J, Wang R, Xie X, Yu X, Pan J, Xu Y, Zheng L. The effect of curcumin on the brain-gut axis in rat model of irritable bowel syndrome: involvement of 5-HT-dependent signaling. Metabolic brain disease. 2015;30(1):47-55.

331. Kawaguchi M, Minamisawa K. Plant–microbe communications for symbiosis. Plant and cell physiology. 2010;51(9):1377-80.

332.   Koranda M, Kaiser C, Fuchslueger L, Kitzler B, Sessitsch A, Zechmeister-Boltenstern S, Richter A. Seasonal variation in functional properties of microbial communities in beech forest soil. Soil Biology and Biochemistry. 2013;60:95-104.

333.   Vicki OA. Declining Nutritional Value of Produce Due to High Yield Selective Seed Breeding: Organic Authority; 2007. Available from: http://www.organicauthority.com/organic-food/organic-food-articles/declining-nutritional-value-of-produce-due-to-high-yield-selective-seed-breeding.html.

334.   Institute W. Crop Yields Expand, but Nutrition Is Left Behind: Worldwatch Institute; 2016. Available from: http://www.worldwatch.org/node/5339.

335.   Bakhøj S, Flint A, Holst JJ, Tetens I. Lower glucose-dependent insulinotropic polypeptide (GIP) response but similar glucagon-like peptide 1 (GLP-1), glycaemic, and insulinaemic response to ancient wheat compared to modern wheat depends on processing. European journal of clinical nutrition. 2003;57(10):1254-61.

336.   Dall M, Calloe K, Haupt-Jorgensen M, Larsen J, Schmitt N, Josefsen K, Buschard K. Gliadin Fragments and a Specific Gliadin 33-mer Peptide Close K ATP Channels and Induce Insulin Secretion in INS-1E Cells and Rat Islets of Langerhans2013.

337.   BAKERpedia. Fermentation: BAKERpedia; 2016. Available from: http://www.bakerpedia.com/processes/fermentation/.

338.   Maioli M, Pes GM, Sanna M, Cherchi S, Dettori M, Manca E, Farris GA. Sourdough-leavened bread improves postprandial glucose and insulin plasma levels in subjects with impaired glucose tolerance. Acta diabetologica. 2008;45(2):91-6.

339.   Greco L, Gobbetti M, Auricchio R, Di Mase R, Landolfo F, Paparo F, Di Cagno R, De Angelis M, Rizzello CG, Cassone A. Safety for patients with celiac disease of baked goods made of wheat flour hydrolyzed during food processing. Clinical Gastroenterology and Hepatology. 2011;9(1):24-9.

340.   Lorenz K, D'Appolonia B. Cereal sprouts: composition, nutritive value, food applications. Critical Reviews in Food Science & Nutrition. 1980;13(4):353-85.

341.   Stevenson L, Phillips F, O'sullivan K, Walton J. Wheat bran: its composition and benefits to health, a European perspective. International journal of food sciences and nutrition. 2012.

342.   Dalla Pellegrina C, Perbellini O, Scupoli MT, Tomelleri C, Zanetti C, Zoccatelli G, Fusi M, Peruffo A, Rizzi C, Chignola R. Effects of wheat germ agglutinin on human gastrointestinal epithelium: insights from an experimental model of immune/epithelial cell interaction. Toxicology and applied pharmacology. 2009;237(2):146-53.

343.   Ruibal-Mendieta NL, Delacroix DL, Mignolet E, Pycke J-M, Marques C, Rozenberg R, Petitjean G, Habib-Jiwan J-L, Meurens M, Quetin-Leclercq J. Spelt (Triticum aestivum ssp. spelta) as a source of breadmaking flours and bran naturally enriched in oleic acid and minerals but not phytic acid. Journal of agricultural and food chemistry. 2005;53(7):2751-9.

344.   Rosén LA, Silva LOB, Andersson UK, Holm C, Östman EM, Björck IM. Endosperm and whole grain rye breads are characterized by low post-prandial insulin response and a beneficial blood glucose profile. Nutrition Journal. 2009;8(1):1.

345.   Lappi J, Mykkänen H, Knudsen KEB, Kirjavainen P, Katina K, Pihlajamäki J, Poutanen K, Kolehmainen M. Postprandial glucose metabolism and SCFA after consuming wholegrain rye bread and wheat bread enriched with bioprocessed rye bran in individuals with mild gastrointestinal symptoms. Nutrition journal. 2014;13(1):1.

346.   Talati R, Baker WL, Pabilonia MS, White CM, Coleman CI. The effects of barley-derived soluble fiber on serum lipids. The Annals of Family Medicine. 2009;7(2):157-63.

347.   Molberg Ø, Uhlen AK, Jensen T, Flæte NS, Fleckenstein B, Arentz–Hansen H, Raki M, Lundin KE, Sollid LM. Mapping of gluten T-cell epitopes in the bread wheat ancestors: implications for celiac disease. Gastroenterology. 2005;128(2):393-401.

348.   van den Broeck H, Hongbing C, Lacaze X, Dusautoir J-C, Gilissen L, Smulders M, van der Meer I. In search of tetraploid wheat accessions reduced in celiac disease-related gluten epitopes. Molecular BioSystems. 2010;6(11):2206-13.

349.   Salentijn EM, Goryunova SV, Bas N, van der Meer IM, van den Broeck HC, Bastien T, Gilissen LJ, Smulders MJ. Tetraploid and hexaploid wheat varieties reveal large differences in expression of alpha-gliadins from homoeologous Gli-2 loci. BMC genomics. 2009;10(1):48.

350.   Benedetti S, Primiterra M, Tagliamonte MC, Carnevali A, Gianotti A, Bordoni A, Canestrari F. Counteraction of oxidative damage in the rat liver by an ancient grain (Kamut brand khorasan wheat). Nutrition. 2012;28(4):436-41.

351. Pelillo M, Iafelice G, Marconi E, Caboni MF. Identification of plant sterols in hexaploid and tetraploid wheats using gas chromatography with mass spectrometry. Rapid communications in mass spectrometry. 2003;17(20):2245-52.

352. Berger A, Jones P, Abumweis SS. Plant sterols: factors affecting their efficacy and safety as functional food ingredients. Lipids Health Dis. 2004;3(5):1-19.

353. Barron J. Benefits & Dangers of Soy Products: Baseline of Health Foundation; 2012. Available from: http://jonbarron.org/article/benefits-dangers-soy-products - .VqHgPEuft8M.

354. Bensky D, ed.; Clavey, Steven, ed.; Stoger, Erich, ed., Gamble, Andrew, ed. Chinese Herbal Medicine: Materia Medica, Third Edition: Eastland Press; 2004.

355. Body Ecology I. How Fermenting Takes the "Allergy" Out of Soy and Other Foods: Body Ecology, Inc.; 2015. Available from: http://bodyecology.com/articles/fermenting_allergy_soy.php.

356. Fallon SaE, Mary G. Tragedy and Hype: The Third International Soy Symposium—Part II 2000. Available from: http://www.tldp.com/issue/11_00/soy.htm.

357. Ishizuki Y, Hirooka Y, Murata Y, Togashi K. [The effects on the thyroid gland of soybeans administered experimentally in healthy subjects]. Nihon Naibunpi Gakkai Zasshi. 1991;67(5):622-9.

358. Divi RL, Doerge DR. Inhibition of thyroid peroxidase by dietary flavonoids. Chemical research in toxicology. 1996;9(1):16-23.

359. Celiac B. Non-Celiac Gluten Sensitivity: Beyond Celiac; 2015. Available from: http://www.beyondceliac.org/celiac-disease/non-celiac-gluten-sensitivity/.

360. Sarah GL. The Real Reason Wheat is Toxic (it's not the gluten): The Healthy Home Economist; 2015. Available from: http://www.thehealthyhomeeconomist.com/real-reason-for-toxic-wheat-its-not-gluten/.

361. Shehata AA, Schrödl W, Aldin AA, Hafez HM, Krüger M. The effect of glyphosate on potential pathogens and beneficial members of poultry microbiota in vitro. Current microbiology. 2013;66(4):350-8.

362. Kau AL, Ahern PP, Griffin NW, Goodman AL, Gordon JI. Human nutrition, the gut microbiome and the immune system. Nature. 2011;474(7351):327-36.

363. Malatesta M, Caporaloni C, Rossi L, Battistelli S, Rocchi MB, Tonucci F, Gazzanelli G. Ultrastructural analysis of pancreatic acinar cells from mice fed on genetically modified soybean. Journal of Anatomy. 2002;201(5):409-15.

364. Mesnage R, Clair E, Gress S, Then C, Székács A, Séralini GE. Cytotoxicity on human cells of Cry1Ab and Cry1Ac Bt insecticidal toxins alone or with a glyphosate-based herbicide. Journal of Applied Toxicology. 2013;33(7):695-9.

365. Aris A, Leblanc S. Maternal and fetal exposure to pesticides associated to genetically modified foods in Eastern Townships of Quebec, Canada. Reproductive Toxicology. 2011;31(4):528-33.

366. Finamore A, Roselli M, Britti S, Monastra G, Ambra R, Turrini A, Mengheri E. Intestinal and peripheral immune response to MON810 maize ingestion in weaning and old mice. Journal of agricultural and food chemistry. 2008;56(23):11533-9.

367. Suskind DL. Nutritional deficiencies during normal growth. Pediatric Clinics of North America. 2009;56(5):1035-53.

368. Zijlmans MA, Korpela K, Riksen-Walraven JM, de Vos WM, de Weerth C. Maternal prenatal stress is associated with the infant intestinal microbiota. Psychoneuroendocrinology. 2015;53:233-45.

369. Douillard J. Perfect Health For Kids: North Atlantic Books; 2004.

370. Carthew P. Safety of carrageenan in foods. Environmental health perspectives. 2002;110(4):A176.

371. Tobacman JK. Review of harmful gastrointestinal effects of carrageenan in animal experiments. Environmental health perspectives. 2001;109(10):983.

372. Chassaing B, Koren O, Goodrich JK, Poole AC, Srinivasan S, Ley RE, Gewirtz AT. Dietary emulsifiers impact the mouse gut microbiota promoting colitis and metabolic syndrome. Nature. 2015;519(7541):92-6.

373. Gitig D. Common food emulsifiers may be linked to metabolic syndrome: Ars Technica; 2015. Available from: http://arstechnica.com/science/2015/02/common-food-emulsifiers-may-be-linked-to-metabolic-syndrome/.

374. Agency CDoFaGR. California's Living Marine Resources: A Status Report: University of California ANR; 2001.

375. Cohen SM, Ito N. A critical review of the toxicological effects of carrageenan and processed eucheuma seaweed on the gastrointestinal tract. CRC Critical Reviews in Toxicology. 2002;32(5):413-44.

376. Bhattacharyya S, O-sullivan I, Katyal S, Unterman T, Tobacman J. Exposure to the common food additive carrageenan leads to glucose intolerance, insulin resistance and inhibition of insulin signalling in HepG2 cells and C57BL/6J mice. Diabetologia. 2012;55(1):194-203.

377. Hennessy M. WhiteWave pulling carrageenan from Silk, Horizon: FoodNavigator-USA.com; 2014. Available from: http://www.foodnavigator-usa.com/Manufacturers/WhiteWave-pulling-carrageenan-from-Silk-Horizon.

378. Erasmus U. Fats That Heal, Fats That Kill. Burnaby, British Columbia, Canada: Books Alive; 1993.

379. Good J. Healthiest Cooking Oil Comparison Chart with Smoke Points and Omega 3 Fatty Acid Ratios: Baseline of Health Foundation; 2012. Available from: http://jonbarron.org/diet-and-nutrition/healthiest-cooking-oil-chart-smoke-points - .VqG7ZUuft8N.

380. LaBaw G, Desrosier N. ANTIBACTERIAL ACTIVITY OF EDIBLE PLANT EXTRACTS a, b. Journal of Food Science. 1953;18(1-6):186-90.

381. A Nogueira-Machado J, M de Oliveira Volpe C. HMGB-1 as a target for inflammation controlling. Recent patents on endocrine, metabolic & immune drug discovery. 2012;6(3):201-9.

382. Zhu S, Li W, Li J, Jundoria A, Sama AE, Wang H. It is not just folklore: the aqueous extract of mung bean coat is protective against sepsis. Evidence-Based Complementary and Alternative Medicine. 2012;2012.

383. Adsule R, Kadam S, Salunkhe D, Luh B. Chemistry and technology of green gram (Vigna radiata [L.] Wilczek). Critical Reviews in Food Science & Nutrition. 1986;25(1):73-105.

384. Service USDoAAR. National Nutrient Database for Standard Reference Release 28: Basic Report: 11043, Mung beans, mature seeds, sprouted, raw: United States Department of Agriculture: Agricultural Research Service; No year listed. Available from: http://ndb.nal.usda.gov/ndb/foods/show/2846?fgcd=&manu=&lfacet=&format=Abridged&count=&max=35&offset=&sort=&qlookup=mung+beans.

385. Chung I-M, Yeo M-A, Kim S-J, Moon H-I. Protective effects of organic solvent fractions from the seeds of Vigna radiata L. wilczek against antioxidant mechanisms. Human & experimental toxicology. 2011;30(8):904-9.

386. Yao Y, Chen F, Wang M, Wang J, Ren G. Antidiabetic activity of Mung bean extracts in diabetic KK-Ay mice. Journal of agricultural and food chemistry. 2008;56(19):8869-73.

387. McIntyre A, Gibson P, Young G. Butyrate production from dietary fibre and protection against large bowel cancer in a rat model. Gut. 1993;34(3):386-91.

388. Canani RB, Costanzo M, Leone L, Pedata M, Meli R, Calignano A. Potential beneficial effects of butyrate in intestinal and extraintestinal diseases. World J Gastroenterol. 2011;17(12):1519-28.

389. Bourdon I, Olson B, Backus R, Richter BD, Davis PA, Schneeman BO. Beans, as a source of dietary fiber, increase cholecystokinin and apolipoprotein B48 response to test meals in men. The Journal of nutrition. 2001;131(5):1485-90.

390. Gershon MD. The Second Brain: A Groundbreaking New Understanding of Nervous Disorders of the Stomach and Intestine: Harper Collins; 1998.

391. Erdman S, Poutahidis T. Probiotic 'glow of health': it's more than skin deep. Beneficial microbes. 2014;5(2):109-19.

392. Neuman H, Debelius JW, Knight R, Koren O. Microbial endocrinology: the interplay between the microbiota and the endocrine system. FEMS microbiology reviews. 2015:fuu010.

393. Gareau MG. Microbiota-gut-brain axis and cognitive function. Microbial Endocrinology: The Microbiota-Gut-Brain Axis in Health and Disease: Springer; 2014. p. 357-71.

394. Erdman SE. Microbes, Oxytocin, and Healthful longevity. Journal of Probiotics & Health.

395. Poutahidis T, Kearney SM, Levkovich T, Qi P, Varian BJ, Lakritz JR, Ibrahim YM, Chatzigiagkos A, Alm EJ, Erdman SE. Microbial symbionts accelerate wound healing via the neuropeptide hormone oxytocin2013.

396. Bercik P, Park A, Sinclair D, Khoshdel A, Lu J, Huang X, Deng Y, Blennerhassett P, Fahnestock M, Moine D. The anxiolytic effect of Bifidobacterium longum NCC3001 involves vagal pathways for gut–brain communication. Neurogastroenterology & Motility. 2011;23(12):1132-9.

397. Diehl GE, Longman RS, Zhang J-X, Breart B, Galan C, Cuesta A, Schwab SR, Littman DR. Microbiota restricts trafficking of bacteria to mesenteric lymph nodes by CX3CR1hi cells. Nature. 2013;494(7435):116-20.

398. Collins SM, Surette M, Bercik P. The interplay between the intestinal microbiota and the brain. Nature Reviews Microbiology. 2012;10(11):735-42.

399. Borre YE, Moloney RD, Clarke G, Dinan TG, Cryan JF. The impact of microbiota on brain and behavior: mechanisms & therapeutic potential. Microbial Endocrinology: The Microbiota-Gut-Brain Axis in Health and Disease: Springer; 2014. p. 373-403.

400. Pert CB, Ruff MR, Weber RJ, Herkenham M. Neuropeptides and their receptors: a psychosomatic network. J immunol. 1985;135(2):820-6.

401. O'Connor A. The Claim: Identical Twins Have Identical DNA: The New York Times; 2008. Available from: http://www.nytimes.com/2008/03/11/health/11real.html?_r=0.

402. Carpenter S. That gut feeling: American Psychological Association; 2012. Available from: http://www.apa.org/monitor/2012/09/gut-feeling.aspx.

403. Dale T. The epigenetic connection: Chiropractic Economics; 2016. Available from: http://www.chiroeco.com/magzine/the-epigenetic-connection/.

404. Hehemann J-H, Correc G, Barbeyron T, Helbert W, Czjzek M, Michel G. Transfer of carbohydrate-active enzymes from marine bacteria to Japanese gut microbiota. Nature. 2010;464(7290):908-12.

405. Liu L, Chen X, Skogerbø G, Zhang P, Chen R, He S, Huang D-W. The human microbiome: a hot spot of microbial horizontal gene transfer. Genomics. 2012;100(5):265-70.

406. Crisp A, Boschetti C, Perry M, Tunnacliffe A, Micklem G. Expression of multiple horizontally acquired genes is a hallmark of both vertebrate and invertebrate genomes. Genome biology. 2015;16(1):50.

407. Smith B. Effect of irritant purgatives on the myenteric plexus in man and the mouse. Gut. 1968;9(2):139-43.

408. U.S. National Library of Medicine NIoh, U.S. Department of Health & Human Services. Drug Record: Cascara (Cascara Sagrada): U.S. National Library of Medicine, National Institutes of health, U.S. Department of Health & Human Services; 2014. Available from: http://livertox.nih.gov/Cascara.htm.

409. Lu K, Chakroborty D, Sarkar C, Lu T, Xie Z, Liu Z, Basu S. Triphala and its active constituent chebulinic acid are natural inhibitors of vascular endothelial growth factor-a mediated angiogenesis. PloS one. 2012;7(8):e43934.

410. Varma SR, Sivaprakasam TO, Mishra A, Kumar LM, Prakash N, Prabhu S, Ramakrishnan S. Protective Effects of Triphala on Dermal Fibroblasts and Human Keratinocytes. PloS one. 2016;11(1).

411. Fujii T, Wakaizumi M, Ikami T, Saito M. Amla (Emblica officinalis Gaertn.) extract promotes procollagen production and inhibits matrix metalloproteinase-1 in human skin fibroblasts. Journal of ethnopharmacology. 2008;119(1):53-7.

412. Chanvorachote P, Pongrakhananon V, Luanpitpong S, Chanvorachote B, Wannachaiyasit S, Nimmannit U. Type I pro-collagen promoting and anti-collagenase activities of Phyllanthus emblica extract in mouse fibroblasts. Journal of cosmetic science. 2009;60(4):395.

413. Watson RR, Zibadi S. Bioactive Dietary Factors and Plant Extracts in Dermatology: Springer; 2013.

414. Slavin J. Fiber and prebiotics: mechanisms and health benefits. Nutrients. 2013;5(4):1417-35.

415. Ke F, Yadav PK, Ju LZ. Herbal medicine in the treatment of ulcerative colitis. Saudi journal of gastroenterology: official journal of the Saudi Gastroenterology Association. 2012;18(1):3.

416. Grieve M. A Modern Herbal: Elm, Slippery: Botanical.com; 2014. Available from: http://botanical.com/botanical/mgmh/e/elmsli09.html.

417. Hage-Sleiman R, Mroueh M, Daher CF. Pharmacological evaluation of aqueous extract of Althaea officinalis flower grown in Lebanon. Pharmaceutical biology. 2011;49(3):327-33.

418. Le Chatelier E, Nielsen T, Qin J, Prifti E, Hildebrand F, Falony G, Almeida M, Arumugam M, Batto J-M, Kennedy S. Richness of human gut microbiome correlates with metabolic markers. Nature. 2013;500(7464):541-6.

419. Foster JA, Neufeld K-AM. Gut–brain axis: how the microbiome influences anxiety and depression. Trends in neurosciences. 2013;36(5):305-12.

420. Mayer EA. Gut feelings: the emerging biology of gut–brain communication. Nature Reviews Neuroscience. 2011;12(8):453-66.

421. Weill Cornell Medical College NY-PH. All About Your GI System: Weill Cornell Medical College, New York-Presbyterian Hospital; No year listed. Available from: http://www.monahancenter.org/screen/all_abo_you.html?name1=All+About+Your+GI+System&type1=2Active.

422. Gopal PK, Prasad J, Gill HS. Effects of the consumption of Bifidobacterium lactis HN019 (DR10 TM) and galacto-oligosaccharides on the microflora of the gastrointestinal tract in human subjects. Nutrition Research. 2003;23(10):1313-28.

423. Danisco. HOWARU® Bifido Probiotics: Danisco; No year listed. Available from: http://www.danisco.com/product-range/probiotics/howarur-premium-probiotics/howarur-bifido-probiotics/.

424. Waller PA, Gopal PK, Leyer GJ, Ouwehand AC, Reifer C, Stewart ME, Miller LE. Dose-response effect of Bifidobacterium lactis HN019 on whole gut transit time and functional gastrointestinal symptoms in adults. Scandinavian journal of gastroenterology. 2011;46(9):1057-64.

425. Douillard J. Perfecting Digestion with Herbs: LifeSpa; 2014. Available from: http://www.lifespa.com/perfecting-digestion-with-herbs/.

426. Douillard J. Euro-Bug Study. 2015.

427. Pollan M. Some of My Best Friends Are Germs: The New York Times Magazine; 2013. Available from: http://www.nytimes.com/2013/05/19/magazine/say-hello-to-the-100-trillion-bacteria-that-make-up-your-microbiome.html?pagewanted=all&_r=0.

428. Carabotti M, Scirocco A, Maselli MA, Severi C. The gut-brain axis: interactions between enteric microbiota, central and enteric nervous systems. Annals of gastroenterology: quarterly publication of the Hellenic Society of Gastroenterology. 2015;28(2):203.

429. Saulnier DM, Ringel Y, Heyman MB, Foster JA, Bercik P, Shulman RJ, Versalovic J, Verdu EF, Dinan TG, Hecht G. The intestinal microbiome, probiotics and prebiotics in neurogastroenterology. Gut microbes. 2013;4(1):17-27.

430. Mayer EA, Knight R, Mazmanian SK, Cryan JF, Tillisch K. Gut microbes and the brain: paradigm shift in neuroscience. The Journal of Neuroscience. 2014;34(46):15490-6.

431. Bercik P, Collins S, Verdu E. Microbes and the gut brain axis. Neurogastroenterology & Motility. 2012;24(5):405-13.

432. Forsythe P, Bienenstock J, Kunze WA. Vagal pathways for microbiome-brain-gut axis communication. Microbial Endocrinology: The Microbiota-Gut-Brain Axis in Health and Disease: Springer; 2014. p. 115-33.

433. Tillisch K, Labus JS. Neuroimaging the Microbiome-Gut-Brain Axis. Microbial Endocrinology: The Microbiota-Gut-Brain Axis in Health and Disease: Springer; 2014. p. 405-16.

434. Rhee SH, Pothoulakis C, Mayer EA. Principles and clinical implications of the brain-gut-enteric microbiota axis. Nature Reviews Gastroenterology and Hepatology. 2009;6(5):306-14.

435. Forsythe P, Kunze WA, Bienenstock J. On communication between gut microbes and the brain. Current opinion in gastroenterology. 2012;28(6):557-62.

436. Downs R, Perna J, Vitelli A, Cook D, Dhurjati P. Model-based hypothesis of gut microbe populations and gut/brain barrier permeabilities in the development of regressive autism. Medical hypotheses. 2014;83(6):649-55.

437. Smith CJ, Emge JR, Berzins K, Lung L, Khamishon R, Shah P, Rodrigues DM, Sousa AJ, Reardon C, Sherman PM. Probiotics normalize the gut-brain-microbiota axis in immunodeficient mice. American Journal of Physiology-Gastrointestinal and Liver Physiology. 2014;307(8):G793-G802.

438. Viaud S, Saccheri F, Mignot G, Yamazaki T, Daillère R, Hannani D, Enot DP, Pfirschke C, Engblom C, Pittet MJ. The intestinal microbiota modulates the anticancer immune effects of cyclophosphamide. Science. 2013;342(6161):971-6.

439. Morse DR, Schacterle GR, Furst L, Zaydenberg M, Pollack RL. Oral digestion of a complex-carbohydrate cereal: effects of stress and relaxation on physiological and salivary measures. The American journal of clinical nutrition. 1989;49(1):97-105.

440. Takahashi M, Fukuda H, Arito H. Brief naps during post-lunch rest: effects on alertness, performance, and autonomic balance. European journal of applied physiology and occupational physiology. 1998;78(2):93-8.

441. Gerson LB. AdvAnces in GeRd. Gastroenterology & hepatology. 2009;5(9):613.

442. Health NP. Heartburn and GERD: Overview: NCBI: PubMed Health; 2015. Available from: http://www.ncbi.nlm.nih.gov/pubmedhealth/PMH0072438/.

443. McCorry LK. Physiology of the autonomic nervous system. American journal of pharmaceutical education. 2007;71(4).

444. Stefano GB, Stefano JM, Esch T. Anticipatory stress response: a significant commonality in stress, relaxation, pleasure and love responses. Medical Science Monitor Basic Research. 2008;14(2):RA17-RA21.

445. Carter CS, Porges SW. The biochemistry of love: an oxytocin hypothesis. EMBO reports. 2013;14(1):12-6.

446. Lehrman NS. Pleasure heals: the role of social pleasure—love in its broadest sense—in medical practice. Archives of internal medicine. 1993;153(8):929-34.

447. Esch T, Stefano GB. The neurobiology of love. Neuroendocrinology Letters. 2005;26(3):175-92.

448. Esch T, Stefano GB. Love promotes health. Neuroendocrinology Letters. 2005;26(3):264-7.

449. Marchant J. Can meditation really slow aging? : CNN; 2014. Available from: http://www.cnn.com/2014/07/10/health/can-meditation-really-slow-aging/index.html.

450. Carroll SB, Prud'Homme B, Gompel N. Regulating evolution. Scientific American. 2008;298(5):60-7.

451. Thomson H. Study of Holocaust survivors finds trauma passed on to children's genes: The Guardian; 2015. Available from: http://www.theguardian.com/science/2015/aug/21/study-of-holocaust-survivors-finds-trauma-passed-on-to-childrens-genes.

452. Thangaswamy S, Bridenbaugh EA, Gashev AA. Evidence of increased oxidative stress in aged mesenteric lymphatic vessels. Lymphatic research and biology. 2012;10(2):53-62.

453. Saketkhoo K, Januszkiewicz A, Sackner MA. Effects of drinking hot water, cold water, and chicken soup on nasal mucus velocity and nasal airflow resistance. CHEST Journal. 1978;74(4):408-10.

454. Ren Y, Ke M, Fang X. Hot Water Swallows May Improve Symptoms in Patients With Achalasia2012.

455. Kauffman Jr G. Gastric mucus and bicarbonate secretion in relation to mucosal protection. Journal of clinical gastroenterology. 1980;3(Suppl 2):45-50.

456. Smith M, Marley K, Seigler D, Singletary K, Meline B. Bioactive properties of wild blueberry fruits. JOURNAL OF FOOD SCIENCE-CHICAGO-. 2000;65(2):352-6.

457. Beekwilder J, Hall RD, Vos R, De C. Identification and dietary relevance of antioxidants from raspberry. Biofactors. 2005;23(4):197-205.

458. Azzini E, Vitaglione P, Intorre F, Napolitano A, Durazzo A, Foddai MS, Fumagalli A, Catasta G, Rossi L, Venneria E. Bioavailability of strawberry antioxidants in human subjects. British journal of nutrition. 2010;104(08):1165-73.

459. John RMSoBM. Red Root: Balance the Body by Way of the Spleen: Redroot Mountain School of Botanical Medicine; 2009. Available from: http://www.redrootmountain.com/red-root-balance-the-body-by-way-of-the-spleen/66.

460. Thorne Research I. Diosmin. Alternative Medicine Review. 2004;9(3).

461. Goto M, Wakagi M, Shoji T, Takano-Ishikawa Y. Oligomeric Procyanidins Interfere with Glycolysis of Activated T Cells. A Novel Mechanism for Inhibition of T Cell Function. Molecules. 2015;20(10):19014-26.

462. Mansouri E, Kooti W, Bazvand M, Boroon MG, Amirzargar A, Afrisham R, Afzalzadeh MR, Ashtary-Larky D, Jalali N. The Effect of Hydro-Alcoholic Extract of Foeniculum vulgare Mill on Leukocytes and Hematological Tests in Male Rats. Jundishapur journal of natural pharmaceutical products. 2015;10(1).

463. Rankin LC, Groom JR, Chopin M, Herold MJ, Walker JA, Mielke LA, McKenzie AN, Carotta S, Nutt SL, Belz GT. The transcription factor T-bet is essential for the development of NKp46+ innate lymphocytes via the Notch pathway. Nature immunology. 2013;14(4):389-95.

464. Georgiev VG, Weber J, Kneschke E-M, Denev PN, Bley T, Pavlov AI. Antioxidant activity and phenolic content of betalain extracts from intact plants and hairy root cultures of the red beetroot Beta vulgaris cv. Detroit dark red. Plant foods for human nutrition. 2010;65(2):105-11.

465. Rao GMM, Rao CV, Pushpangadan P, Shirwaikar A. Hepatoprotective effects of rubiadin, a major constituent of Rubia cordifolia Linn. Journal of ethnopharmacology. 2006;103(3):484-90.

466. Tripathi Y, Sharma M. Comparison of the antioxidant action of the alcoholic extract of Rubia cordifolia with rubiadin. Indian journal of biochemistry & biophysics. 1998;35(5):313-6.

467. Kurien BT, Harris VM, Quadri SM, Coutinho-de Souza P, Cavett J, Moyer A, Ittiq B, Metcalf A, Ramji HF, Truong D. Significantly reduced lymphadenopathy, salivary gland infiltrates and proteinuria in MRL-lpr/lpr mice treated with ultrasoluble curcumin/turmeric: increased survival with curcumin treatment. Lupus science & medicine. 2015;2(1):e000114.

468. Da W, Zhu J, Wang L, Sun Q. Curcumin suppresses lymphatic vessel density in an in vivo human gastric cancer model. Tumor Biology. 2015:1-9.

469. Jattujan P, Pinlaor S, Charoensuk L, Arunyanart C, Welbat JU, Chaijaroonkhanarak W. Curcumin prevents bile canalicular alterations in the liver of hamsters infected with Opisthorchis viverrini. The Korean journal of parasitology. 2013;51(6):695-701.

470. Gohil KJ, Patel JA, Gajjar AK. Pharmacological review on Centella asiatica: a potential herbal cure-all. Indian journal of pharmaceutical sciences. 2010;72(5):546.

471. Benzie I, Wachtel-Galor, S., editors. Herbal Medicine: Biomolecular and Clinical Aspects. 2nd edition. Benzie I, Wachtel-Galor, S., editors, editor. Boca Raton, FL: CRC Press/Taylor & Francis; 2011.

472. Pitsch F. Recent guidelines in chronic venous disease: the place of Daflon 500 mg. Phlebolymphology. 2011;18(1):24-9.

473. Bergan JJ, Schmid-Schönbein GW, Takase S. Therapeutic approach to chronic venous insufficiency and its complications: place of Daflon® 500 mg. Angiology. 2001;52(1 suppl):S43-S7.

474. Smith P. Neutrophil activation and mediators of inflammation in chronic venous insufficiency. Journal of vascular research. 1999;36(Suppl. 1):24-36.

475. Korthuis RJ, Gute DC. Anti-inflammatory actions of a micronized, purified flavonoid fraction in ischemia/reperfusion. FlaVonoids in Cell Function: Springer; 2002. p. 181-90.

476. Jean T, Bodinier MC. Mediators involved in inflammation: effects of Daflon 500 mg on their release. Angiology. 1994;45(6 Pt 2):554-9.

477. Valensi P, Behar A, De Champvallins M, Attalah M, Boulakia F, Attali JR. Effects of a purified micronized flavonoid fraction on capillary filtration in diabetic patients. Diabetic medicine. 1996;13(10):882-8.

478. Valensi P, Behar A. Clinical implications of impaired microcirculation. International angiology: a journal of the International Union of Angiology. 1995;14(3 Suppl 1):26-31.

479. Behar A, Valensi P, de Champvallins M, Cohen Boulakia F, Albagli B. Capillary filtration and lymphatic resorption in diabetes. Application to the pharmacodynamic activity of Daflon 500 mg. International angiology: a journal of the International Union of Angiology. 1988;8(4 Suppl):27-9.

480. Buckshee K, Takkar D, Aggarwal N. Micronized flavonoid therapy in internal hemorrhoids of pregnancy. International Journal of Gynecology & Obstetrics. 1997;57(2):145-51.

481. Cospite M. Double-blind, placebo-controlled evaluation of clinical activity and safety of Daflon 500 mg in the treatment of acute hemorrhoids. Angiology. 1994;45(6 Pt 2):566-73.

482. Nazıroğlu M, Güler M, Özgül C, Saydam G, Küçükayaz M, Sözbir E. Apple cider vinegar modulates serum lipid profile, erythrocyte, kidney, and liver membrane oxidative stress in ovariectomized mice fed high cholesterol. The Journal of membrane biology. 2014;247(8):667-73.

483. Johnston CS, Gaas CA. Vinegar: medicinal uses and antiglycemic effect. Medscape General Medicine. 2006;8(2):61.

484. Estaki M, DeCoffe D, Gibson DL. Interplay between intestinal alkaline phosphatase, diet, gut microbes and immunity. World journal of gastroenterology: WJG. 2014;20(42):15650.

485. Dawson-Hughes B, Harris SS, Ceglia L. Alkaline diets favor lean tissue mass in older adults. The American journal of clinical nutrition. 2008;87(3):662-5.

486. Schwalfenberg GK. The alkaline diet: is there evidence that an alkaline pH diet benefits health? Journal of Environmental and Public Health. 2011;2012.

487. Coates G, O'Brodovich H, Jefferies A, Gray G. Effects of exercise on lung lymph flow in sheep and goats during normoxia and hypoxia. Journal of Clinical Investigation. 1984;74(1):133.

488. Downey HF, Durgam P, Williams Jr AG, Rajmane A, King HH, Stoll ST. Lymph flow in the thoracic duct of conscious dogs during lymphatic pump treatment, exercise, and expansion of extracellular fluid volume. Lymphatic research and biology. 2008;6(1):3-13.

489. Nedergaard M. Brain Drain. Scientific American. March 2016:P. 45-9.

490. Myers J. Exercise and cardiovascular health. Circulation. 2003;107(1):e2-e5.

491. Olszewski W, Engeset A, Icger P, Sokolowski J, Theodorsen L. Flow and composition of leg lymph in normal men during venous stasis, muscular activity and local hyperthermia. Acta Physiologica Scandinavica. 1977;99(2):149-55.

492. Iyengar BKS. Light on Yoga: The Classic Guide to Yoga by the World's Foremost Authority: Harper Collins Publishers; 2006.

244 | EAT WHEAT

493. Marciani L, Cox E, Hoad C, Totman JJ, Costigan C, Singh G, Shepherd V, Chalkley L, Robinson M, Ison R. Effects of various food ingredients on gallbladder emptying. European journal of clinical nutrition. 2013;67(11):1182-7.
494. Douillard J. The Colorado Cleanse, Third Edition: LifeSpa Products, LLC; 2013.
495. Rana SS, Bhasin DK, Sharma V, Rao C, Gupta R, Singh K. Role of endoscopic ultrasound in evaluation of unexplained common bile duct dilatation on magnetic resonance cholangiopancreatography. Annals of gastroenterology: quarterly publication of the Hellenic Society of Gastroenterology. 2013;26(1):66.
496. Turumin J, Shanturov V, Turumina H. The role of the gallbladder in humans. Rev Gastroenterol Mex. 2013;78(03):177-87.
497. Kasicka-Jonderko A, Jonderko K, Gajek E, Piekielniak A, Zawislan R. SLUGGISH GALLBLADDER EMPTYING AND GASTROINTESTINAL TRANSIT AFTER INTAKE OF COMMON ALCOHOLIC BEVERAGES. JPP. 2014(02):06.
498. Kasicka-Jonderko A, Jonderko K, Bożek M, Kamińska M, Mgłosiek P. Potent inhibitory effect of alcoholic beverages upon gastrointestinal passage of food and gallbladder emptying. Journal of gastroenterology. 2013;48(12):1311-23.
499. Cohen B. Auburn's Secret Sauce: Beet Juice: The Wall Street Journal; 2014. Available from: http://www.wsj.com/articles/auburns-secret-sauce-beet-juice-1410978433.
500. Presley TD, Morgan AR, Bechtold E, Clodfelter W, Dove RW, Jennings JM, Kraft RA, King SB, Laurienti PJ, Rejeski WJ. Acute effect of a high nitrate diet on brain perfusion in older adults. Nitric Oxide. 2011;24(1):34-42.
501. Murphy M, Eliot K, Heuertz RM, Weiss E. Whole beetroot consumption acutely improves running performance. Journal of the Academy of Nutrition and Dietetics. 2012;112(4):548-52.
502. Webb AJ, Patel N, Loukogeorgakis S, Okorie M, Aboud Z, Misra S, Rashid R, Miall P, Deanfield J, Benjamin N. Acute blood pressure lowering, vasoprotective, and antiplatelet properties of dietary nitrate via bioconversion to nitrite. Hypertension. 2008;51(3):784-90.
503. Kahlon T, Chapman M, Smith G. In vitro binding of bile acids by okra, beets, asparagus, eggplant, turnips, green beans, carrots, and cauliflower. Food chemistry. 2007;103(2):676-80.
504. Váli L, Stefanovits-Bányai É, Szentmihályi K, Fébel H, Sárdi É, Lugasi A, Kocsis I, Blázovics A. Liver-protecting effects of table beet (Beta vulgaris var. rubra) during ischemia-reperfusion. Nutrition. 2007;23(2):172-8.
505. Udupa A, Nahar P, Shah S, Kshirsagar M, Ghongane B. A Comparative Study of Effects of Omega-3 Fatty Acids, Alpha Lipoic Acid and Vitamin E in Type 2 Diabetes Mellitus. Annals of medical and health sciences research. 2013;3(3):442-6.
506. Eisele TA. Determination of D-malic acid in apple juice by liquid chromatography: collaborative study. Journal of AOAC International. 1995;79(1):50-4.
507. Russell I, Michalek JE, Flechas JD, Abraham GE. Treatment of fibromyalgia syndrome with Super Malic: a randomized, double blind, placebo controlled, crossover pilot study. The Journal of rheumatology. 1995;22(5):953-8.
508. Rodgers AL, Webber D, de Charmoy R, Jackson GE, Ravenscroft N. Malic acid supplementation increases urinary citrate excretion and urinary pH: implications for the potential treatment of calcium oxalate stone disease. Journal of Endourology. 2014;28(2):229-36.
509. Reddy RR, Srinivasan K. Dietary fenugreek and onion attenuate cholesterol gallstone formation in lithogenic diet–fed mice. International journal of experimental pathology. 2011;92(5):308-19.
510. Kashyap LaD, Vadiya Bhagwan. Materia Medica of Ayurveda. New Delhi: Concept Publishing Company; 2000.
511. Visser S. Effect of humic substances on mitochondrial respiration and oxidative phosphorylation. Science of the Total Environment. 1987;62:347-54.
512. Carrasco-Gallardo C, Guzmán L, Maccioni RB. Shilajit: a natural phytocomplex with potential procognitive activity. International Journal of Alzheimer's Disease. 2012;2012.
513. Boonjaraspinyo S, Boonmars T, Aromdee C, Puapairoj A, Wu Z. Indirect effect of a turmeric diet: enhanced bile duct proliferation in Syrian hamsters with a combination of partial obstruction by Opisthorchis viverrini infection and inflammation by N-nitrosodimethylamine administration. Parasitology research. 2011;108(1):7-14.

514. Bested AC, Logan AC, Selhub EM. Intestinal microbiota, probiotics and mental health: from Metchnikoff to modern advances: Part II-contemporary contextual research. Gut Pathog. 2013;5(3):1-14.

515. Shoba G, Joy D, Joseph T, Majeed M, Rajendran R, Srinivas P. Influence of piperine on the pharmacokinetics of curcumin in animals and human volunteers. Planta med. 1998;64(4):353-6.

516. Cole GM, Teter B, Frautschy SA. Neuroprotective effects of curcumin. The molecular targets and therapeutic uses of curcumin in health and disease: Springer; 2007. p. 197-212.

517. Yang F, Lim GP, Begum AN, Ubeda OJ, Simmons MR, Ambegaokar SS, Chen PP, Kayed R, Glabe CG, Frautschy SA. Curcumin inhibits formation of amyloid β oligomers and fibrils, binds plaques, and reduces amyloid in vivo. Journal of Biological Chemistry. 2005;280(7):5892-901.

518. Kulkarni S, Dhir A, Akula KK. Potentials of curcumin as an antidepressant. The Scientific World Journal. 2009;9:1233-41.

519. Ramakrishna Rao R, Platel K, Srinivasan K. In vitro influence of spices and spice-active principles on digestive enzymes of rat pancreas and small intestine. Food/Nahrung. 2003;47(6):408-12.

520. Oso AO, Awe AW, Awosoga FG, Bello FA, Akinfenwa TA, Ogunremi EB. Effect of ginger (Zingiber officinale Roscoe) on growth performance, nutrient digestibility, serum metabolites, gut morphology, and microflora of growing guinea fowl. Tropical animal health and production. 2013;45(8):1763-9.

521. Satyanarayana S, Sushruta K, Sarma G, Srinivas N, Raju GS. Antioxidant activity of the aqueous extracts of spicy food additives-evaluation and comparison with ascorbic acid in in vitro systems. Journal of herbal pharmacotherapy. 2004;4(2):1-10.

522. O Mahony R, Al-Khtheeri H, Weerasekera D, Fernando N, Vaira D, Holton J, Basset C. Bactericidal and anti-adhesive properties of culinary and medicinal plants against Helicobacter pylori. World Journal of Gastroenterology. 2005;11(47):7499.

523. Valussi M. Functional foods with digestion-enhancing properties. International journal of food sciences and nutrition. 2012;63(sup1):82-9.

524. Platel K, Srinivasan K. Stimulatory influence of select spices on bile secretion in rats. Nutrition Research. 2000;20(10):1493-503.

525. Bhaswant M, Poudyal H, Mathai ML, Ward LC, Mouatt P, Brown L. Green and black cardamom in a diet-induced rat model of metabolic syndrome. Nutrients. 2015;7(9):7691-707.

526. System PPSDI. Coriandrum sativum Linn.: Pharma Professional Services: Drug Information System; 2014. Available from: http://druginfosys.com/herbal/Herb.aspx?Code=155&Name=Coriandrum sativum Linn.&type=1.

527. System PPSDI. Cuminum cyminum Linn.: Pharma Professional Services: Drug Information System; 2014. Available from: http://druginfosys.com/herbal/Herb.aspx?Code=160&name=Cuminum cyminum Linn.&type=1.

528. System PPSDI. Foeniculum vulgare Miller: Pharma Professional Services: Drug Information System; 2014. Available from: http://druginfosys.com/herbal/Herb.aspx?Code=171&name=Foeniculum vulgare Miller&type=1.

529. Johri R, Zutshi U. An Ayurvedic formulation 'Trikatu'and its constituents. Journal of ethnopharmacology. 1992;37(2):85-91.

530. Choudhury R, Kumar A, Reddy A, Garg A. Thermal neutron activation analysis of essential and trace elements and organic constituents in Trikatu: An Ayurvedic formulation. Journal of Radioanalytical and Nuclear Chemistry. 2007;274(2):411-9.

531. Jain V, Saraf S, Saraf S. Spectrophotometric Determination of Piperine in Trikatu Churna: An Ayurvedic Formulation. Asian Journal of Chemistry. 2007;19(7):5331.

532. Shailajan S, Sayed N, Joshi H, Tiwari B. Standardization of an Ayurvedic formulation-Trikatu Churna using bioanalytical tools2011.

533. Paul Choudhury R, Kumar A, Garg A, Reddy A. Thermal neutron activation analysis of essential and trace elements in Trikatu: an ayurvedic prescription. Application of radiotracers in chemical, environmental and biological sciences V 22006.

534. Jain V, Vyas A, Saraf S, Saraf S. HPLC Determination of Piperine in 'Trikatu Churna'a Potent Ayurvedic Formulation for Routine Quality Control. Asian Journal of Research in Chemistry. 2011;4(2):183-6.

535. Meena A, Mangal A, Simha G, Rao M, Panda P, Singh H, Padhi M, Babu R. Evaluation of Phamacognostic and Physicochemical Parameters of Trikatu churna-an Ayurvedic Classical Drug. Research Journal of Pharmacy and Technology. 2011;4(12):1882-4.

536.   Kusters JG, van Vliet AH, Kuipers EJ. Pathogenesis of Helicobacter pylori infection. Clinical microbiology reviews. 2006;19(3):449-90.

537.   Control CfD, Prevention. Awareness of prediabetes--United States, 2005-2010. MMWR Morbidity and mortality weekly report. 2013;62(11):209.

538.   Prevention CfDCa. New CDC Diabetes Report: Centers for Disease Control and Prevention; 2014. Available from: http://www.cdc.gov/media/dpk/2014/dpk-diabetes-report.html.

539.   Cai Z, Liu N, Wang C, Qin B, Zhou Y, Xiao M, Chang L, Yan L-J, Zhao B. Role of RAGE in Alzheimer's disease. Cellular and molecular neurobiology. 2015:1-13.

540.   Yamagishi S-i, Nakamura N, Suematsu M, Kaseda K, Matsui T. Advanced Glycation End Products: A Molecular Target for Vascular Complications in Diabetes. Molecular Medicine. 2015;21(Suppl 1):S32.

541.   Bangert A, Andrassy M, Müller A-M, Bockstahler M, Fischer A, Volz CH, Leib C, Göser S, Korkmaz-Icöz S, Zittrich S. Critical role of RAGE and HMGB1 in inflammatory heart disease. Proceedings of the National Academy of Sciences. 2016;113(2):E155-E64.

542.   Jahan H, Choudhary MI. Glycation, carbonyl stress and AGEs inhibitors: a patent review. Expert opinion on therapeutic patents. 2015;25(11):1267-84.

543.   Data SN. Nutrition Facts: Wheat flour, white, all-purpose, enriched, bleached: SELF Nutrition Data; 2014. Available from: http://nutritiondata.self.com/facts/cereal-grains-and-pasta/5745/2.

544.   Einkorn.com. Types of Wheat: Nutritional Content & Health Benefits Comparison: Einkorn.com; 2015. Available from: http://www.einkorn.com/types-of-wheat-nutritional-content-health-benefits-comparison/.

545.   Thorup A, Gregersen S, Jeppesen PB. Ancient Wheat Diet Delays Diabetes Development in a Type 2 Diabetes Animal Model. The review of diabetic studies: RDS. 2013;11(3-4):245-57.

546.   Yamaguchi N, Sugita R, Miki A, Takemura N, Kawabata J, Watanabe J, Sonoyama K. Gastrointestinal Candida colonisation promotes sensitisation against food antigens by affecting the mucosal barrier in mice. Gut. 2006;55(7):954-60.

547.   Kumamoto CA. Inflammation and gastrointestinal Candida colonization. Current opinion in microbiology. 2011;14(4):386-91.

548.   Pizzo G, Giuliana G, Milici M, Giangreco R. Effect of dietary carbohydrates on the in vitro epithelial adhesion of Candida albicans, Candida tropicalis, and Candida krusei. The new microbiologica. 2000;23(1):63-71.

549.   Vargas SL, Patrick C, Ayers G, Hughes W. Modulating effect of dietary carbohydrate supplementation on Candida albicans colonization and invasion in a neutropenic mouse model. Infection and immunity. 1993;61(2):619-26.

550.   Ipatenco S. How Much Sugar Is Really in a Soda? : SF Gate; No year listed. Available from: http://healthyeating.sfgate.com/much-sugar-really-soda-4922.html.

551.   Corporation S. Vanilla Latte: Starbucks Corporation; 2016. Available from: http://www.starbucks.com/menu/drinks/espresso/vanilla-latte.

552.   Company NJ. Green Machine: Naked Juice Company; 2016. Available from: http://www.nakedjuice.com/our-products/juice/green-machine.

553.   Krasowska A, Murzyn A, Dyjankiewicz A, Łukaszewicz M, Dziadkowiec D. The antagonistic effect of Saccharomyces boulardii on Candida albicans filamentation, adhesion and biofilm formation. FEMS yeast research. 2009;9(8):1312-21.

554.   Ogbolu D, Oni A, Daini O, Oloko A. In vitro antimicrobial properties of coconut oil on Candida species in Ibadan, Nigeria. Journal of medicinal food. 2007;10(2):384-7.

555.   Suez J, Korem T, Zeevi D, Zilberman-Schapira G, Thaiss CA, Maza O, Israeli D, Zmora N, Gilad S, Weinberger A. Artificial sweeteners induce glucose intolerance by altering the gut microbiota. Nature. 2014;514(7521):181-6.

556.   Low YQ, Lacy K, Keast R. The role of sweet taste in satiation and satiety. Nutrients. 2014;6(9):3431-50.

557.   Douillard J. Weight Balancing eBook: LifeSpa.com; 2016. Available from: http://lifespa.com/ayurvedic-weight-loss-ebook/.

558.   Bjørnholt JV, Erikssen G, Aaser E, Sandvik L, Nitter-Hauge S, Jervell J, Erikssen J, Thaulow E. Fasting blood glucose: an underestimated risk factor for cardiovascular death. Results from a 22-year follow-up of healthy nondiabetic men. Diabetes care. 1999;22(1):45-9.

559.   Becker D. Highest Quality Supplements Since 1980. Cancer.4:20-9.

560. Crane PK, Walker R, Hubbard RA, Li G, Nathan DM, Zheng H, Haneuse S, Craft S, Montine TJ, Kahn SE. Glucose levels and risk of dementia. New England Journal of Medicine. 2013;369(6):540-8.

561. News B. Why do people put on differing amounts of weight? : BBC News; 2016. Available from: http://www.bbc.com/news/magazine-35193414.

562. Chrościcki P, Usarek M, Bryla J. [The role of biological clock in glucose homeostasis]. Postepy higieny i medycyny doswiadczalnej (Online). 2012;67:569-83.

563. Mattson MP, Allison DB, Fontana L, Harvie M, Longo VD, Malaisse WJ, Mosley M, Notterpek L, Ravussin E, Scheer FA. Meal frequency and timing in health and disease. Proceedings of the National Academy of Sciences. 2014;111(47):16647-53.

564. Hatori M, Vollmers C, Zarrinpar A, DiTacchio L, Bushong EA, Gill S, Leblanc M, Chaix A, Joens M, Fitzpatrick JA. Time-restricted feeding without reducing caloric intake prevents metabolic diseases in mice fed a high-fat diet. Cell metabolism. 2012;15(6):848-60.

565. Chaix A, Zarrinpar A, Miu P, Panda S. Time-restricted feeding is a preventative and therapeutic intervention against diverse nutritional challenges. Cell metabolism. 2014;20(6):991-1005.

566. Garaulet M, Gómez-Abellán P, Alburquerque-Béjar JJ, Lee Y-C, Ordovás JM, Scheer FA. Timing of food intake predicts weight loss effectiveness. International journal of obesity. 2013;37(4):604-11.

567. Oike H, Oishi K, Kobori M. Nutrients, clock genes, and chrononutrition. Current nutrition reports. 2014;3(3):204-12.

568. Lui Z-J, Chu H-H, Wu Y-C, Yang S-K. Effect of two-step time-restricted feeding on the fattening traits in geese. Asian-Australasian journal of animal sciences. 2014;27(6):841.

569. Douillard J. The 3-Season Diet. New York: Harmony Books; 2001.

570. Bellisle F, McDevitt R, Prentice AM. Meal frequency and energy balance. British Journal of Nutrition. 1997;77(S1):S57-S70.

571. Doheny K. 'Grazing' vs. Standard Meals for Weight Loss: WebMD.com; 2014. Available from: http://www.webmd.com/diet/20140327/grazing-appears no better for weight loss than standard-meals.

572. Michaels J. MYTH: Constant Grazing Boosts Your Metabolism: Jillian Michaels; No year listed. Available from: http://www.jillianmichaels.com/fit/lose-weight/myth-small-meals.

573. News B. Syndrome X the 'silent killer': BBC News; 2002. Available from: http://news.bbc.co.uk/2/hi/health/1933706.stm.

574. Kshirsagar SG. YOU SHOULD IGNORE THIS TERRIBLE PIECE OF POPULAR DIETING ADVICE: Tips on Healthy Living from Simon & Schuster; 2015. Available from: http://www.tipsonhealthyliving.com/diet-and-fitness/you-should-ignore-this-terrible-piece-of-popular-dieting-advice.

575. Herron RE, Fagan JB. Lipophil-mediated reduction of toxicants in humans: an evaluation of an ayurvedic detoxification procedure. Alternative therapies in health and medicine. 2002;8(5):40-51.

576. Douillard J. Body, Mind, and Sport: The Mind-Body Guide to Lifelong Health, Fitness, and Your Personal Best: Harmony; 2001; Rev. Upd. edition.

577. Lehrer PM, Gevirtz R. Heart rate variability biofeedback: how and why does it work? Frontiers in psychology. 2014;5.

578. Martin D, Rehder K, Parker J, Taylor A. High-frequency ventilation: lymph flow, lymph protein flux, and lung water. Journal of Applied Physiology. 1984;57(1):240-5.

579. Pal G, Velkumary S. Effect of short-term practice of breathing exercises on autonomic functions in normal human volunteers. Indian Journal of Medical Research. 2004;120(2):115.

580. Bhutkar MV, Bhutkar PM, Taware GB, Surdi AD. How effective is sun salutation in improving muscle strength, general body endurance and body composition? Asian journal of sports medicine. 2011;2(4):259.

581. Bhavanani AB, Udupa K, Madanmohan P. A comparative study of slow and fast suryanamaskar on physiological function. International journal of yoga. 2011;4(2):71.

582. Godse AS, Shejwal BR, Godse AA. Effects of suryanamaskar on relaxation among college students with high stress in Pune, India. International journal of yoga. 2015;8(1):15.

583. Sinha AN, DeePAK D, Gusain VS. Assessment of the effects of pranayama/alternate nostril breathing on the parasympathetic nervous system in young adults. Journal of clinical and diagnostic research: JCDR. 2013;7(5):821.

584. Meerman R, Brown AJ. When somebody loses weight, where does the fat go? BMJ. 2014;349:g7257.

585. Tanaka Y, Morikawa T, Honda Y. An assessment of nasal functions in control of breathing. Journal of Applied Physiology. 1988;65(4):1520-4.

586. Stuart CA, Howell ME, Baker JD, Dykes RJ, Duffourc MM, Ramsey MW, Stone MH. Cycle training increased GLUT4 and activation of mTOR in fast twitch muscle fibers. Medicine and science in sports and exercise. 2010;42(1):96.

587. Nevill M, Holmyard D, Hall G, Allsop P, Van Oosterhout A, Burrin J, Nevill A. Growth hormone responses to treadmill sprinting in sprint-and endurance-trained athletes. European journal of applied physiology and occupational physiology. 1996;72(5-6):460-7.

588. Cryan JF, O'Mahony S. The microbiome-gut-brain axis: from bowel to behavior. Neurogastroenterology & Motility. 2011;23(3):187-92.

589. Stetka BSaY, Kit. Why We Shop: The Neuropsychology of Consumption: Medscape; 2014. Available from: http://www.medscape.com/viewarticle/814649_2.

590. Volkow ND, Wang G-J, Baler RD. Reward, dopamine and the control of food intake: implications for obesity. Trends in cognitive sciences. 2011;15(1):37-46.

591. Scheele D, Wille A, Kendrick KM, Stoffel-Wagner B, Becker B, Güntürkün O, Maier W, Hurlemann R. Oxytocin enhances brain reward system responses in men viewing the face of their female partner. Proceedings of the National Academy of Sciences. 2013;110(50):20308-13.

592. Uvnäs-Moberg K, Handlin L, Petersson M. Self-soothing behaviors with particular reference to oxytocin release induced by non-noxious sensory stimulation. Frontiers in psychology. 2014;5.

593. Uvnas-Moberg K, Petersson M. Oxytocin, a mediator of anti-stress, well-being, social interaction, growth and healing. Z Psychosom Med Psychother. 2005;51(1):57-80.

594. Morhenn V, Beavin LE, Zak PJ. Massage increases oxytocin and reduces adrenocorticotropin hormone in humans. Altern Ther Health Med. 2012;18(6):11-8.

595. Shamay-Tsoory SG, Abu-Akel A, Palgi S, Sulieman R, Fischer-Shofty M, Levkovitz Y, Decety J. Giving peace a chance: oxytocin increases empathy to pain in the context of the Israeli–Palestinian conflict. Psychoneuroendocrinology. 2013;38(12):3139-44.

596. Matthiesen AS, Ransjö-Arvidson AB, Nissen E, Uvnäs-Moberg K. Postpartum maternal oxytocin release by newborns: effects of infant hand massage and sucking. Birth. 2001;28(1):13-9.

597. Fredrickson BL, Grewen KM, Coffey KA, Algoe SB, Firestine AM, Arevalo JM, Ma J, Cole SW. A functional genomic perspective on human well-being. Proceedings of the National Academy of Sciences. 2013;110(33):13684-9.

598. Sci-News.com Ea. Positive Psychology Influences Gene Expression in Humans, Scientists Say: Sci-News.com; 2013. Available from: http://www.sci-news.com/othersciences/psychology/science-positive-psychology-gene-expression-humans-01305.html.

599. Fredrickson BL, Grewen KM, Algoe SB, Firestine AM, Arevalo JM, Ma J, Cole SW. Psychological Well-Being and the Human Conserved Transcriptional Response to Adversity. PloS one. 2015;10(3):e0121839.

600. Jeste DV, Palmer BW, Rettew DC, Boardman S. Positive psychiatry: its time has come. The Journal of clinical psychiatry. 2015;76(6):1,478-683.

601. Kubzansky LD, Mendes WB, Appleton A, Block J, Adler GK. Protocol for an experimental investigation of the roles of oxytocin and social support in neuroendocrine, cardiovascular, and subjective responses to stress across age and gender. BMC Public Health. 2009;9(1):481.

602. Knowles SR, Nelson EA, Palombo EA. Investigating the role of perceived stress on bacterial flora activity and salivary cortisol secretion: a possible mechanism underlying susceptibility to illness. Biological psychology. 2008;77(2):132-7.

603. Bosch J, de Geus EJ, Ligtenberg TJ, Nazmi K, Veerman EC, Hoostraten J, Amerongen, AV. Salivary MUC5B-mediated adherence (ex vivo) of Helicobacter pylori during acute stress. Psychosomatic Medicine. 2000;62(1):40-9.

604. Keightley PC, Koloski NA, Talley NJ. Pathways in gut-brain communication: Evidence for distinct gut-to-brain and brain-to-gut syndromes. Australian and New Zealand Journal of Psychiatry. 2015;49(3):207-14.

605. Konturek P, Brzozowski, T, Konturek SJ. Stress and the gut: pathophysiology, clinical consequences, diagnostic approach and treatment options. Physiol Pharmacol. 2011;62(6):591-9.

Appendices

Appendix A
SEASONAL GROCERY LISTS

SPRING GROCERY LIST
(March–June)

- Eat **more** foods that are **Pungent (Spicy), Bitter, Astringent / Light, Dry, Warm**: Such as flavorful steamed veggies, brothy soups, brown rice.
- Eat **less** foods that are Sweet, Sour, Salty / Heavy, Cold, Oily: Such as fried foods, ice cream, heavy dairy, breads.
- **Curious about a food not on this list?** Taste it. If it has 2 of the 3 spring tastes (pungent/spicy, bitter, astringent), it is balancing. Prepare it in a way that is light, dry and/or warm.

Choose Organic and non-GMO when possible.
Eat more of your favorite foods from this list.

An asterisk means that this food is a Spring Superfood.
If you like it, eat more of it.

251

Vegetables

*Alfalfa Sprouts	*Chilies, dried	*Lettuce
Artichokes	Cilantro	*Mushrooms
*Asparagus	*Collard Greens	*Mustard Greens
*Bean Sprouts	*Corn	*Onions
Beets	*Dandelion	*Parsley
*Bell Peppers	*Endive	*Peas
*Bitter Melon	Fennel	*Potatoes, baked
Broccoli	*Garlic	*Radishes
*Brussels Sprouts	Ginger	Seaweed
*Cabbage	*Green Beans	Snow Peas
*Carrots	*Hot Peppers	*Spinach
*Cauliflower	Jicama	*Swiss Chard
*Celery	*Kale	*Turnips Watercress
*Chicory	Leeks	

Fruit

Eat fruit separately from other foods.

Apples	Lemons, Limes	Raspberries
Blueberries	Papayas	Strawberries
*Dried Fruit (all)	Pears	All Berries
Grapefruit	Pomegranates (sour)	

Dairy

Favor raw or vat-pasteurized.

Ghee (moderation)	(moderation)	*Goat milk
Low-fat yogurt	Rice/Soy milk	

Oils

Flax	Coconut Oil
Hemp	

Sweeteners

Favor natural whole foods sweeteners, in moderation:

*Honey - Raw	Maple Syrup	Molasses

Herbs & Spices

Anise	Coriander	Oregano
Asafoetida	Cumin	Peppermint
Basil	Dill	Poppy Seeds
Bay Leaf	Fennel	Rosemary
*Black Pepper	Fenugreek	Saffron
Chamomile	Garlic	Sage
Caraway	Ginger	Spearmint
Cardamom	Horseradish	Thyme
*Cayenne	Marjoram	Turmeric
Cinnamon	Mustard	
*Clove	Nutmeg	

Condiments

Carob	Pickles

Legumes

*All Sprouted Beans	Fava	*Mung
Adzuki	*Kidney	Split Pea
Black Gram	*Lentils	
Garbanzo	*Lima	

Lean Meat & Fish

Chicken	Ocean fish *(moderation)*
Duck *(moderation)*	Turkey
Eggs *(moderation)*	
Freshwater fish	
Lamb *(moderation)*	

Nuts & Seeds

Filberts	Pumpkin
Pinons	Sunflower

Whole Grains

Amaranth	Corn	Quinoa
Barley	Millet	Rice, Brown, long grain
Buckwheat	Oats, dry	Rye

Herb Tea

Alfalfa	*Cloves	*Orange Peel
*Cardamom	*Dandelion	*Strawberry Leaf
*Chicory	*Ginger	
*Cinnamon	*Hibiscus	

Beverages

Black Tea *(moderation)*	*(moderation)*
Coffee	Water *(room temp. to hot)*

SUMMER GROCERY LIST

(July–October)

- Eat **more** foods that are **Sweet, Bitter, Astringent / Cool, Heavy, Oily**: Such as salads, smoothies, and fresh fruit.
- Eat **less** foods that are Pungent (Spicy), Sour, Salty / Hot, Light, Dry: Such as spicy foods, hot beverages.
- **Curious about a food not on this list?** Taste it. If it has 2 of the 3 summer tastes (sweet, bitter, astringent), it is balancing. Prepare it in a way that is cool, heavy and/or oily.

Choose Organic and non-GMO when possible.
Eat more of your favorite foods from this list.

An asterisk means that this food is a Summer Superfood.
If you like it, eat more of it.

Vegetables

Alfalfa Sprouts

*Artichokes

*Asparagus

Avocados

Bean Sprouts

*Beet greens

*Bell Peppers

*Bitter Melon

*Broccoli

*Cabbage

*Cauliflower

*Celery

Chicory

*Cilantro

Collard Greens

Corn

*Cucumbers

*Dandelion

Eggplant

Endive

*Fennel

Green Beans

*Jicama

*Kale

*Lettuce

Mushrooms

Mustard Greens

*Okra

Parsley

Peas

Pumpkin

*Radishes (moderation)

*Seaweed

*Snow Peas

Spinach (moderation)

*Squash, Acorn

Squash, Winter

Sweet Potatoes

Swiss Chard

Tomatoes (sweet)

Turnip Greens

*Watercress

*Zucchini

Fruit

Eat fruit separately from other foods.

*Apples

*Apricots

*Blueberries

*Cantaloupe

*Cherries (ripe)

*Cranberries

Dates

Dried Fruit

Figs

*Grapes

*Guavas

*Mangoes

*Melon (all)

Nectarines

Oranges (sweet)

Papayas (small amounts)

*Peaches (ripe and/or peeled)

*Pears

*Persimmons

*Pineapple (sweet)

*Plums (ripe)

*Pomegranates (sour)

*Raspberries

*Strawberries

Tangerines (sweet)

Meats

Beef (moderation)	Eggs (moderation)	Pork
Chicken	Freshwater Fish	Shrimp (moderation)
Duck (moderation)	Lamb (moderation)	Turkey

Legumes

*Adzuki	*Garbanzo	*Mung
Bean Sprouts	Kidney	*Split Pea
*Black Gram	Lentils	*Tofu
*Fava	Lima	

Condiments

Carob	Mayonnaise

Oils

Almond	*Coconut	*Olive
Avocado	Flax	Ghee

Herbs & Spices

Anise	*Coriander	Peppermint
Asafoetida	Cumin	Saffron
*Chamomile	Fennel	Spearmint

Whole Grains

*Barley	*Rice	Wheat
Oat	Rye	

Tea

*Chicory	*Hibiscus
*Dandelion	*Mint

Beverages

Water (room temp or cool)

Sweeteners

Favor natural whole foods sweeteners, in moderation:

Maple Syrup (small amounts)	Raw Sugar
	Rice Syrup

Nuts & Seeds

Almonds	Macadamias	*Sunflower
*Coconut	Pine Nuts	
Flax	*Pumpkin	

Dairy

Favor raw and vat-pasteurized.	Cheese (moderation)	Ice Cream
	Cottage Cheese	*Milk
Butter	*Ghee	
*Rice/Soy Milk		

WINTER GROCERY LIST

(November–February)

- Eat **more** foods that are **Sweet, Sour, Salty / Heavy, Oily, Moist, Hot**: Such as soups, stews, steamed veggies, and more fat and protein.

- Eat **less** foods that are Pungent (Spicy), Bitter, Astringent / Light, Cold, Dry: Such as salads, smoothies, cold foods and beverages, crackers, chips and salsa.

- **Curious about a food not on this list?** Taste it. If it has 2 of the 3 winter tastes (sweet, sour and salty), it is balancing. Prepare it in a way that is moist, oily, heavy and/or warm.

Choose Organic and non-GMO when possible.
Eat more of your favorite foods from this list.

An asterisk means that this food is a Winter Superfood.
If you like it, eat more of it.

Vegetables

Cook all vegetables and add a healthy oil, such as ghee, and warming spices. Favor root vegetables:

Artichokes, hearts	Eggplant, cooked	Potatoes, mashed
*Avocados	*Garlic	*Pumpkins
*Beets	Ginger	Seaweed, cooked
*Brussels Sprouts	Hot Peppers	Squash, Acorn
*Carrots	Leeks	*Squash, Winter
*Chilies	Okra	*Sweet Potatoes
Corn	Onions	*Tomatoes
Fennel	Parsley	Turnips

Oils

Most (healthy) oils:

*Almond	*Flax	*Safflower
*Avocado	*Mustard	*Sesame
*Canola	*Olive	Sunflower
*Coconut	*Peanut	

Fruit

Favor sweet, sour or heavy fruits. Eat fruit separately from other foods. Serve warm:

Apples, cooked	*Grapes	Pineapples
Apricots	Guava	Plums
*Bananas	*Lemons	Strawberries
Blueberries	*Limes	*Tangerines
Cantaloupe, with lemon	*Mangoes	
Cherries	Nectarines	
Coconuts, ripe	*Oranges	
Cranberries, cooked	*Papayas	
*Dates	Peaches	
*Figs	Pears, ripe	
*Grapefruit	*Persimmons	

Meat & Fish
All meat, eggs and fish are good:

*Beef	*Fish, freshwater & ocean	*Shrimp
*Chicken	*Lamb	*Turkey
*Crabs	*Lobster	*Venison
*Duck	*Oysters	
*Eggs	*Pork	

Spices
Most spices and herbs are good:

*Anise	Coriander	Oregano
*Asafoetida	*Cumin	Peppermint
*Basil	Dill	Poppy Seeds
Bay Leaf	*Fennel	Rosemary
*Black Pepper	Fenugreek	*Saffron
Caraway	Garlic	Sage
*Cardamom	*Ginger	Spearmint
Cayenne	Horseradish	Tarragon
Chamomile	Marjoram	Thyme
*Cinnamon	Mustard	*Turmeric
Clove	Nutmeg	

Condiments
Favor sweet, sour and salty tastes:

Carob	Lemon or Lime	*Salt
Dulse	Mayonnaise	Vinegar
Fermented foods	Pickles	

Nuts & Seeds
Most nuts and seeds are good:

*Almonds	Coconuts	Lotus Seed
*Brazil Nuts	*Filberts	*Macadamias
*Cashews	*Flax	*Peanuts, raw

*Pecans   *Pistachios   *Walnuts

*Pinons   Sunflower

Dairy

All dairy is good, ideally at room temperature or warm (such as boiled milk). Favor raw or vat-pasteurized.

*Butter	*Cream	Non-Dairy substitutes
*Buttermilk	*Ghee	Sour Cream
*Cheese	*Kefir	Yogurt
*Cottage cheese	Milk, not cold	

Sweeteners

Most natural whole foods sweeteners, in moderation:

Honey - Raw	*Molasses	*Rice Syrup
*Maple Syrup	Sugar, Raw	

Legumes

Mung—split, yellow   Tofu

Beverages

Favor warm-hot drinks that are low in caffeine and alcohol:

Alcohol (moderation)	Coffee (moderation)
Black Tea (moderation)	Water (warm or hot)

Herb Teas

Choose warming and/or calming teas, such as:

*Cardamom	*Cinnamon	*Ginger
*Chamomile	*Cloves	*Orange Peel

Whole Grains

Most grains are good. Best eaten warm, moist and with a healthy oil:

*Amaranth	Millet (moderation)	*Quinoa
Buckwheat (moderation)	*Oats	Rice

*Rice, Brown
Rye (moderation)
*Wheat

Appendix B
HOMEMADE SOURDOUGH BREAD RECIPES

Sourdough Bread: The Old World Way

This is a traditional recipe given to me by my mother who, while living in Europe many years ago, received it from the daughter of traditional bakers in Lourdes, France. The baker's daughter lovingly wrote it down on a napkin during one of their visits, and told my mother that it had been passed down from generation to generation.

⟫⟫ Making the Starter ⟪⟪
(takes 1–3 weeks)

 Tip: Don't be intimidated by the fact the starter takes 1–3 weeks to make. You only need to make the starter the very first time you make bread, as the starter can be refortified and used for years.

Ingredients:
- Whole wheat flour (Rye flour, or organic all-purpose flour may be used, but use the same type throughout the process.)
- Filtered water
- 1 teaspoon raw, organic honey

Directions:

1. In a 4 cup glass container, mix about 1/4 cup lukewarm pure, filtered water and 1/2 cup whole wheat flour—enough to create a mixture similar to the consistency of medium batter.

2. Stir in 1 teaspoon of raw, organic honey.

3. Cover with a piece of cloth or plastic wrap and let sit for 24 hours in a dry, warm place.

4. After 24 hours, add a little bit more water and flour (roughly 3 tablespoons of each). This is known as it's "feeding." Stir well, cover, and let it sit for another 24 hours.

5. On the 3rd day, during the second feeding, remove 1/2 of the starter (can be used for making pancakes) and add 1/4 cup of lukewarm pure, filtered water and 1/2 cup of flour to the other half. Mix well and let sit until mixture bubbles and doubles in size—up to 3 days.

6. Once the mixture has doubled in size and is bubbly, remove 50 percent of it and store half in the refrigerator to make future starter and feed the other half as before.

7. It should take only 12 hours by now for the mixture to double in size.

8. Do not use the starter until it is at least 1 week old, and until it can double itself between feedings. (You can continue the same "50 percent refrigerate, 50 percent feed" procedure up to 3 months, but it should be ripe and ready to use after 1 week. For the fullest sourdough flavor, it is best to use your first starter after 3 weeks of feeding.)

⟫⟫ Making Sourdough Bread ⟪⟪
(Lourdes, France Recipe)

Tip: This process takes about 16 hours, including resting the dough overnight. Plan accordingly.

Ingredients:

- 1/4 cup starter (recipe above)
- 1 1/2 cups whole wheat flour

- 2 cups organic all-purpose flour
- 1 1/2 cups filtered water
- 2 teaspoons salt

Directions:

1. In the evening, mix together 1 1/2 cups whole wheat flour and 2 cups organic all-purpose flour in a large glass or ceramic bowl.
2. Then dissolve 1/4 cup of your starter into 1 1/2 cups pure, filtered water, and add to the flour mixture. Stir until well mixed. Mixture should be thick, similar to pancake batter.
3. Cover bowl with a piece of thick cloth or plastic wrap and let sit until morning (12–18 hours is even better). Keep the temperature of dough and the room around 70°F or warmer. Add a blanket to keep it warm if needed.
4. The next day, place dough onto a lightly floured surface and sprinkle 2 teaspoons salt onto the dough along with a light dusting of a bit more all-purpose flour and knead for a minute to incorporate the salt thoroughly.
5. Gently flatten dough out with hands to make what looks like a large square-ish pancake. Then fold in both outer 1/3 sides onto the center third; you should have 3 layers. Now, fold the dough in half, so that you have 6 layers of dough.
6. Cover this dough-mound loosely with a damp cloth and let it rest for 15 minutes.
7. With lightly flour-dusted hands, roll dough into a ball and transfer dough onto a kitchen cloth that is well-floured. Cover with another cloth and /or light blanket, and let rise its final time for about 2–6 hours, depending on the temperature of the room and weather.
8. Score the top of the dough with a knife 3–4 times. Just before baking.
9. Bake in covered La Cloche or Dutch oven preheated to 500°F for 30 minutes.
10. Remove cover and reduce heat to 450°F and bake an additional 15 minutes.

11. Enjoy! It's tasty *and* supports your health. Nothing beats home-baked bread, made with fresh, whole food ingredients and love!

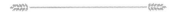

KRIPALU ORGANIC ARTISAN SOURDOUGH RECIPE

The following recipe is from the head baker, Cathy Ligenza at the Kripalu Center for Yoga and Health in Lenox, Massachusetts. She has been baking bread since she was a teenager and her bread is the best I have tasted—made with all organic ingredients with no additives or oils.

 Reminder: Learning to bake sourdough bread is as much an art as it is a science. It is nothing like throwing some brownie mix in the oven. Consider this a form of therapy and allow yourself to fall in love this age-old process. Enjoy…

Of course, the first concern is ingredients. Find the best organic whole grain and all-purpose or bread flour, flax seed and the purest salt you can find. Not all salt is equal! She uses Himalayan in the bakery, but also likes Celtic, Icelandic and some Mediterranean Sea Salts. Flours will vary from time to time, even from the same source, depending upon the harvest and the age of the wheat. In other words, be flexible in your sourcing of flours as long as they are organic and whole grain. If you must use unfiltered chlorinated water, it will not affect the activity of your bread drastically, but ideally you will use the best water you can, at least filtered.

Sourdough starter is flour, water and yeast and bacteria. No matter what method you use to initiate your first starter, it will always incorporate the yeast and friendly bacteria (think probiotic—pro-living) thriving in your environment. You can purchase the initial starter online or you can make your own from scratch. There are many recipes online. She has made a delicious starter using a method of Nancy Silverton's of La Brea Bakery, utilizing the yeast naturally occurring on grapes and the ambient yeast and bacteria in the environment. She has also made wonderful starter with just flour and water. After a starter is established, it needs to be refrigerated and fed regularly with fresh water and flour to keep it vital. She feeds hers every 3 days. To use as leavening, it needs to show vitality; that is, when fed, it doubles within 4–8 hours, depending upon the temperature. It can be used as leavening, to make the bread rise, at that point, or refrigerated to ripen and used within 5 days. If the starter is refrigerated over 5 days, you can re-feed it until it is nice and active again. When to use is based upon preference of flavor and your own schedule. Once you are comfortable with the process, there is some flexibility in each step!

The sourdough starter used at Kripalu is around a century old, originally brought back from Belgium, by Richard Bourdain of Berkshire Mountain Bakery.

⟫⟫ Cathy's Sourdough, Sunflower Flax Bread ⟪⟪
Two 2 pound loaves requires two 9" x 5" bread pans

Ingredients:
- Starter
- Water
- All-purpose flour
- 2/3 cup sunflower seeds
- 2/3 cup flax seeds
- 1 cup whole wheat flour
- 3 tablespoons rye flour
- 1 tablespoon salt

Directions:
Step One:
Refresh your starter… up until 5 days before making bread in fridge.
To make 1 pound starter, begin with:
- 1/4 cup of your starter (2 ounces)
- 3/4 cup water (6 ounces)
- 8 ounces all-purpose flour

Mix these ingredients until well incorporated and allowed to rise until it doubles in size, which can take 4–8 hours. It is a soft dough consistency that is easy to handle and becomes somewhat wetter after it rises. This starter is now ready to use or it can sit for up to 5 days in the refrigerator before using. The longer it sits in the refrigerator, the stronger your starter will be and the sourer your sourdough bread will become.

Step Two: Soak the Seeds

- 2/3 cup sunflower seeds (3 ounces)
- 2/3 cup flax seeds (3 ounces)
- 3/4 cup water (6 ounces)

Soak seeds in water overnight.

Step Three: Making the Bread Dough

- 4 1/4 cups all-purpose bread flour (1 pound 6 ounces)
- 1 cup whole-wheat flour (6 ounces)
- 3 tablespoons rye flour (1 ounce)

Put these dry ingredients into mixing bowl with the already soaked seeds.

Next, you will need:

- 2 1/3 cups water (1 pound 3 ounces)
- 3/4 cup starter (6 ounces)
- 1 tablespoon salt (.6 ounces)

Gradually add and mix in the water into the dry ingredients, withholding a bit of it at the point when a dough forms. Mix in the starter. Stir/knead in to incorporate. Let rest 20 minutes. This important step allows the starter to start working before any other additions.

Step Four: Add the Salt

At this point you will be deciding how much more water to add, and this is something that you will know once you've made a few loaves. A wetter dough makes a moister bread. But if it is too wet, it won't have the structure to rise well. Start with the quantity in this recipe and if you want, adjust if you know or sense the bread needs it. Otherwise, keep with the recipe until you have a feel for the process. Variables are ambient humidity, moisture of the flours, and your starter.

Salt inhibits microbial growth. Wet the salt with the remaining water and mix/knead the salted water into dough and knead until smooth and elastic. This is gluten in action. You will absolutely know when it is smooth and elastic. The subsequent rising action of the dough will have a further smoothing out of the gluten, so better to under-knead than to over-knead. If using a mixer, use a low speed. Slow and gentle is the rule. Place the dough in an oiled bowl, brush with a little more oil to prevent from drying, cover the bowl and allow to rise. Depending on the temperature and humidity of your environment, this can take from 1–3 hours. Unless you are bound by time concerns, there is no benefit to hurrying this process. You will know when the bread has finished its first rise by its texture. When pulled slightly, you will feel between your fingers that the dough contains bubbles of gas. It no longer feels like a heavy piece of putty; you can feel the lightness and liveliness of the yeast/bacterial activity. The clump of dough you are pulling on will be somewhat warm and will willingly stretch and pull, showing that more gluten development has occurred.

Step Five: Refrigerate the Dough

Turn the dough out and cut into 2 equal pieces. Form into loaves and place into lightly greased pans. If the dough rose slowly, the loaves can be left out to begin rising for an hour or so before refrigerating where they will slowly rise and develop in flavor. If they rose very fast, it's best to refrigerate them immediately. Leave refrigerated 8–16 hours, your choice.

Step Six: Final Rise

Pull out to rise until they rise up, look a bit puffy and you see bubbles starting to form under the skin. Again, this depends upon time and humidity. Feel free to do what you can to adjust these factors at this point. Cathy likes a warm and humid final rise, though sometimes the rising is too far advanced to submit to any further encouragement. But since heat in fermentation is a factor in the breaking down of phytic acid in whole grains and seeds, she generally gladly utilizes it.

Step Seven: Bake Your Bread

Place in preheated 425° oven, misting the tops of the loaves and the oven to prevent the initial formation of a crust. The bubbles of gas are expanding due to the sudden heat, which cause the loaves to expand. If a crust forms too fast, the bread cannot expand to its maximum capacity. A pan of hot water placed in the oven while preheating helps as well. Mist again a couple of times during the first 10 minutes, and again shortly before removing from the oven, and you will have a beautiful crust. The bread will be done in about 45 minutes, depending upon your preference in doneness and your oven.

This recipe can be adjusted to suit your needs in as many ways as you can imagine.

If you find yourself making sourdough bread on a regular basis, you might want to look into investing in a wooden breadbox! Your bread will keep over a week and be perfectly moist and delicious.

Note: I would like to thank Cathy for sharing her recipe with us. Learning how to bake healthy bread is a rare skill and Cathy is an expert that is rare these days in a world of mass produced foods.

Appendix C
AYURVEDIC SUPERFOOD KITCHARI RECIPE

⁓⁓⁓ **Kitchari Recipe** ⁓⁓⁓

Ingredients:

 Tip: For best results, use all organic ingredients.

- 1 cup split yellow mung dahl beans
- 1 cup white long grain rice *(quinoa or millet can be used as alternatives)*
- 8 cups of water *(or 4 cups vegetable broth and 4 cups water)*
- 2-3 tablespoons of grass-fed ghee
- 1 tablespoon ginger, freshly grated
- 1/2 teaspoon turmeric powder *(or 1 teaspoon freshly grated)*
- 1/2 teaspoon coriander powder *(or 1 teaspoon seeds)*
- 1/2 teaspoon cumin powder *(or 1 teaspoon seeds)*
- 1/2 teaspoon whole cumin seeds *(or 1/4 teaspoon powdered)*

- 1/2 teaspoon brown or yellow mustard seeds
- 1 pinch hing, also known as asafoetida *(optional)*
- 1/2 teaspoon salt
- 1 small handful fresh cilantro leaves, chopped

Directions:
1. Rinse split yellow mung dahl beans and rice *(or alternative)* together a few times, until water is less murky.
2. Toast the spices *(optional):* Heat a heavy skillet over medium heat. Add spices and toast 2–5 minutes or until spices are fragrant and lightly browned, stirring constantly to prevent burning. Remove from heat.
3. In a large saucepan, combine rice *(or alternative),* beans, water, and spices. Add 2–3 tablespoons of grass-fed ghee.

 Tip: When using kitchari during cleansing, as in the *Short Home Cleanse*, omit the ghee.

4. Cover and bring to a boil. Reduce heat to low and simmer until rice *(or alternative)* and beans are soft (at least 30 minutes, longer is ideal). If time permits, you can cook it longer by adding more water. Your goal is kitchari that is well-cooked and soupy.
5. Garnish with salt and cilantro, and enjoy!

Appendix D

SUN SALUTATION
YOGA INSTRUCTIONS

SUN SALUTATION

The "sun salute" is a complete Ayurvedic exercise also known as *Surya Namaskara*. This series of postures simultaneously integrates the whole physiology including mind, body, and breath. It strengthens and stretches all the major muscle groups, lubricates the joints, conditions the spine, massages the internal organs and increases blood flow and circulation. Traditionally, it is a cycle of 12 postures performed in a fluid sequence one right after another. Each motion should be synchronized with the breath. Alternatively, you may want to try giving each posture time to activate the movement of prana (energy) by staying in each posture with deep nasal breathing for 1–2 minutes.

If you are new to yoga, I highly recommend taking a few classes with an experienced teacher to ensure that you have the proper alignment. If in doubt, move slowly and be gentle with yourself and your ability. You do not need to do the poses perfectly to benefit.

Perform Sun Salutations for a minimum of 12 minutes each day, or follow my Everyday Yoga programs on the Gaiam DVDs: *Ayurveda for Detox, Ayurveda for Stress Relief* or *Ayurveda for Weight Loss.*

How to do Sun Salutation

1. Salutation

Normal, restful breathing

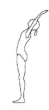

2. Raised Arms

Inhale

3. Hand to Foot

Exhale

4. Equestrian

Inhale

5. Mountain

Exhale

6. Eight Limbs

No breathing

7. Cobra

Inhale

8. Mountain

Exhale

9. Equestrian

Inhale

10. Hand to Foot

Exhale

11. Raised Arms

Inhale

12. Salutation

Exhale

Sun Salutation: Standing Chair Modification

You will need a sturdy, straight-backed chair for this exercise. Be sure to place the back of the chair against a wall to ensure sturdiness.

 Reminder: Pain is always an indication that you are pushing too hard. You will reap the most benefits by relaxing into these postures, rather than straining through them.

1. Stand with a straight back facing the seat of the chair, with feet close together but not touching. Bring your palms together in front of your chest. *Standing prayer pose.*

2. Interlace your thumbs and stretch your arms straight out in front of you, parallel to the ground. Let your gaze follow your hands as you reach them up overhead, stretching and elongating the spine from its base at the tailbone all the way up to the fingertips. *Mountain pose.*

3. Keeping your arms by your ears and your gaze towards your hands, hinge forward at the hips and soften your knees to a slight bend. When you come to a natural pause, place your hands on the seat of the chair and relax your head down. *Forward bend.*

4. Bending your right knee, reach your left foot back and place it a few feet behind you on the floor. Keep your left leg straight and your right leg bent at the knee. Look up. *Left side lunge.*

5. Keeping both palms on the chair and the right knee bent, lower your left knee to the ground. Arch your back, gently squeezing your shoulder blades together and opening your chest, and look up. *Kneeling left side lunge.*

6. Reach your right knee back to meet the left so that both knees are on the floor and the feet are together. Pushing into your palms, straighten your legs back. Gaze towards your feet and gently stretch heels back towards the ground. *Modified downward-facing dog.*

7. Keep arms and legs in place. With a straight back, tilt head slightly and look up. *Halfway lift.*

8. Bend your left knee and step the left foot forward a few feet to its original position. Keep the right leg stretched straight out behind you. Look up. *Right side lunge.*

9. Bend right knee to the floor. Then arch your back, gently squeezing your shoulder blades together and opening your chest, and look up. *Kneeling right side lunge.*

10. Your palms still on the chair, step your right foot up to meet the left and straighten your legs. *Forward fold.*

11. Interlace your thumbs and stretch your arms out, letting your gaze follow your hands as you reach them up overhead, stretching and elongating the spine from its base at the tailbone all the way to the fingertips. *Mountain pose.*

12. Slowly lower your arms down and bring your palms together in front of your chest. Relax, breathe, and be with your body for a few moments, taking note of how you feel. *Standing prayer pose.*

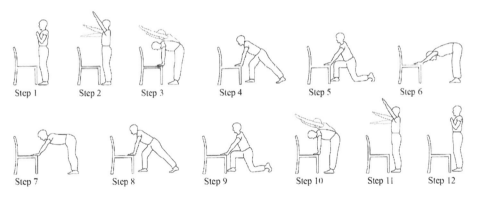

Step 1   Step 2   Step 3   Step 4   Step 5   Step 6
Step 7   Step 8   Step 9   Step 10   Step 11   Step 12

Repeat exercise 3 times (as long as there is no pain)

SUN SALUTATION: SEATED CHAIR MODIFICATION
You will need a sturdy, straight-backed chair for this exercise.

Reminder: Pain is always an indication that you are pushing too hard. You will reap the most benefits by relaxing into these postures, rather than straining through them.

1. Sit with a straight back with your legs together. If your feet do not reach the floor, put a pillow below your feet so they do not dangle. Bring your palms together in front of your chest. *Seated prayer pose.*

2. Interlace your thumbs and stretch your arms straight out in front of you, parallel to the ground. Gaze towards your hands as you reach them up overhead, stretching and elongating the spine from its base at the tailbone, all the way up to your fingertips. *Seated extended mountain pose.*

3. Keep your arms near your ears and keep gazing at your hands as you slowly hinge forward at the hips. When you come to a natural pause, let your head relax towards your thighs and gently bring your arms towards the ground. *Forward fold.*

4. With both hands, take hold of your right leg behind the knee and gently lift up. Bring your torso forward towards your right thigh as far as is comfortable. *Seated right side lunge.*

5. Continuing to hold your right leg up, arch your back, gently squeezing your shoulder blades together and opening your chest. Look up. *Halfway lift.*

6. Lengthen the back of your neck, bringing your head back to a neutral position, and gently release your right leg. Interlace your thumbs and stretch your arms straight out in front of you. Keeping your gaze directly on your hands, slowly hinge forward at the hips. When you come to a natural pause, let your head relax towards your thighs and gently bring your arms towards the ground. *Forward fold.*

7. With a straight back, bring your torso to an upright position. Rest your palms on your thighs with your fingers pointing towards your knees and elbows bent. Arch your back, gently squeezing your shoulder blades together and opening your chest, and let your head tilt back slightly. Look up. *Seated mountain pose.*

8. Lengthen the back of your neck, bringing your head back to a neutral position. With both hands, take hold of your left leg behind the knee. Gently lift up. Bring your torso forward towards your left thigh as far as comfortable. *Seated left side lunge.*

9. Continuing to hold your left leg up, arch your back, sliding your shoulder blades towards one another across your back and opening your chest. Look up. *Halfway lift.* Lengthen the back of your neck, bringing your head back to center, and gently release your left leg.

10. Interlace your thumbs and stretch your arms straight out in front of you. Keeping your gaze on your hands, slowly hinge forward at the hips. When you come to a natural pause, let your head relax towards your thighs and gently bring your arms towards the ground. *Forward fold.*

11. Interlace your thumbs and stretch your arms out, gazing at your hands as you reach them up overhead, stretching and elongating the spine from its base at the tailbone, all the way up to your fingertips. *Seated extended mountain pose.*

12. Slowly lower your arms down and bring your palms together in front of your chest. Relax your hands to your lap. Breathe and relax your body for a few moments, taking note of how you feel. *Seated prayer pose.*

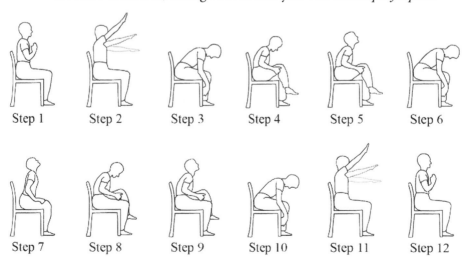

Step 1   Step 2   Step 3   Step 4   Step 5   Step 6

Step 7   Step 8   Step 9   Step 10   Step 11   Step 12

Repeat exercise 3 times (as long as there is no pain)

PRODUCTS AND SERVICES
AT LIFESPA.COM

Free Video-Newsletter

lifespa.com/newsletter

This 3x weekly video-newsletter unites ancient wisdom and modern science to tackle some of the most controversial health topics today. Over 700 free articles and videos are available online to help you achieve your personal health goals.

Online Store

store.lifespa.com

LifeSpa offers only the highest quality herbs, nutritional supplements and products to support you on your journey towards optimal health. Our interactive website helps you understand which herbs or supplements will be best for you.

Free eBooks

lifespa.com/ebooks

Dr. John's library of free eBooks is a robust repositiory of transformational knowledge. These include but aren't limited to the Ayurvedic Weight Balancing eBook, the Blood Sugar Secrets for Health & Longevity eBook, the Short Home

Cleanse eBook and the Protein Solution: Combat Hidden Signs of Protein Deficiency eBook.

What is Your Ayurvedic Body Type and Skin Type?

lifespa.com/healthquiz

Take one of our free interactive quizzes to learn how you can stay balanced and healthy with the best foods, herbs and lifestyle practices for your body type.

ABOUT THE AUTHOR

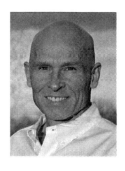

Dr. John Douillard, DC, CAP, is a globally recognized leader in the fields of natural health, Ayurveda, and sports medicine. He is the creator of LifeSpa.com, the leading Ayurvedic health and wellness resource on the web with over 700 natural health and fitness articles and videos proving ancient wisdom with modern science. Dr. John is the former Director of Player Development and nutrition counselor for the New Jersey Nets NBA team, author of 6 books, a repeat guest on the Dr. Oz show, and featured in *Woman's World* Magazine, *Huffington Post*, *Yoga Journal* and dozens of other national publications. He directs LifeSpa, the 2013 Holistic Wellness Center of the year in Boulder, CO.

INDEX

CPSIA information can be obtained
at www.ICGtesting.com
Printed in the USA
LVOW08s1739070217
523493LV00006B/1275/P